THE FOOT STRENGTH PLAN

HEALTHY FEET, THE TRUTH ABOUT ORTHOTICS, AND MORE

COLIN DOMBROSKI, PHD

To my family:
You are my inspiration.
I love you all very much
(to the moon and dinosaurs).

ISBN (paperback): 978-1-7772376-1-5
ISBN (ebook): 978-1-7772376-0-8

Cover design by Aaniyah Ahmed
Interior design and production by Domini Dragoone
Photography by One-12 Photography
Chapter opening images sourced from 123rf.com

DISCLAIMER

This book is intended to supply general educational information only. This book is not intended to be used as a substitute for professional medical advice. Each patient is unique, and solutions and their results vary. Users should execute the exercises in this book with professional advice from a qualified physician or foot specialist.

Any mention of specific companies, organizations, or authorities in this book does not imply endorsement by the author or publisher, nor does the mention of specific companies, organizations, or authorities imply that those entities endorse this book, its author, or the publisher.

Any third-party sites linked to this book are not under the author's control. The author is not responsible for anything on the linked sites, including—without limitation—any content, links to other sites, any changes to those sites, or any policies concerning those sites. The author provides links as a convenience only, and such links do not imply endorsement by the author or publisher, nor does mention of specific companies, organizations, or authorities imply that those entities endorse this book, its author, or the publisher.

For bonuses, videos of exercises, a list of references, and more, visit www.stuffaboutfeet.com

CONTENTS

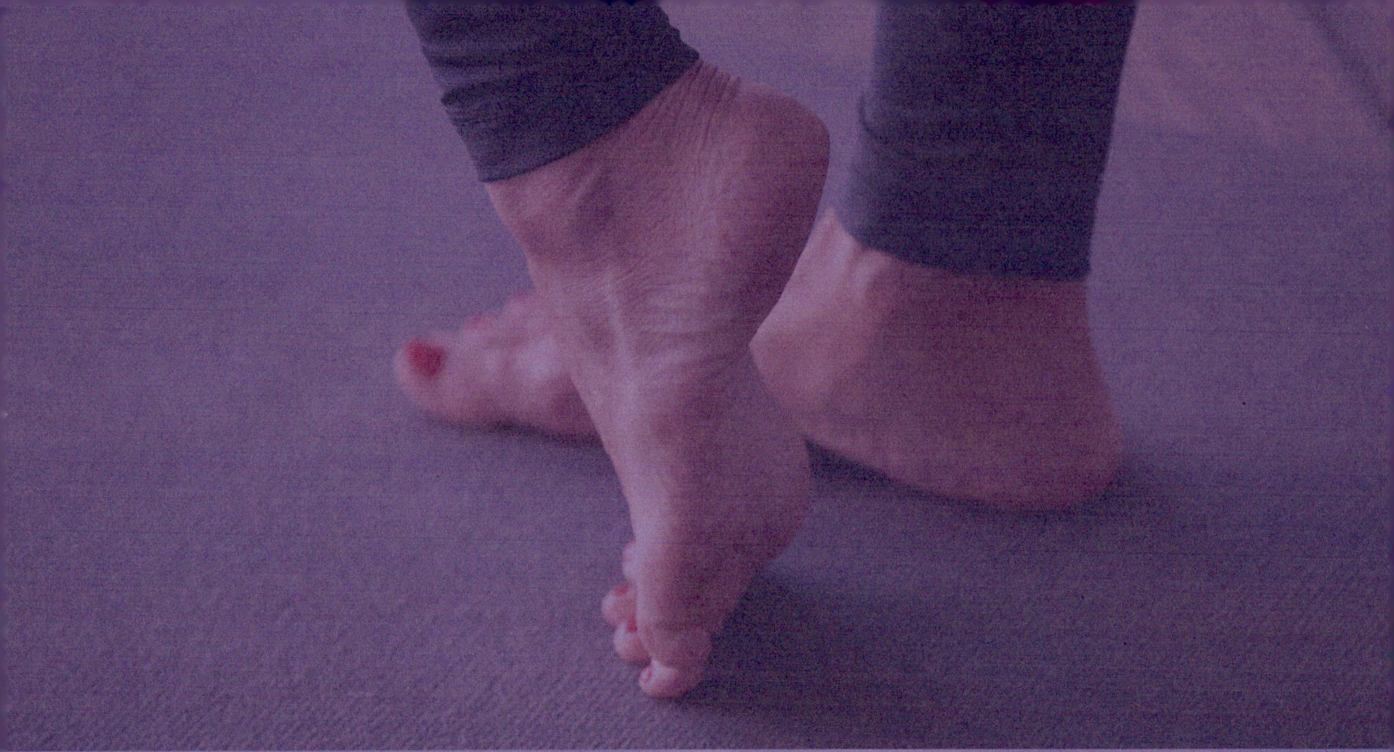
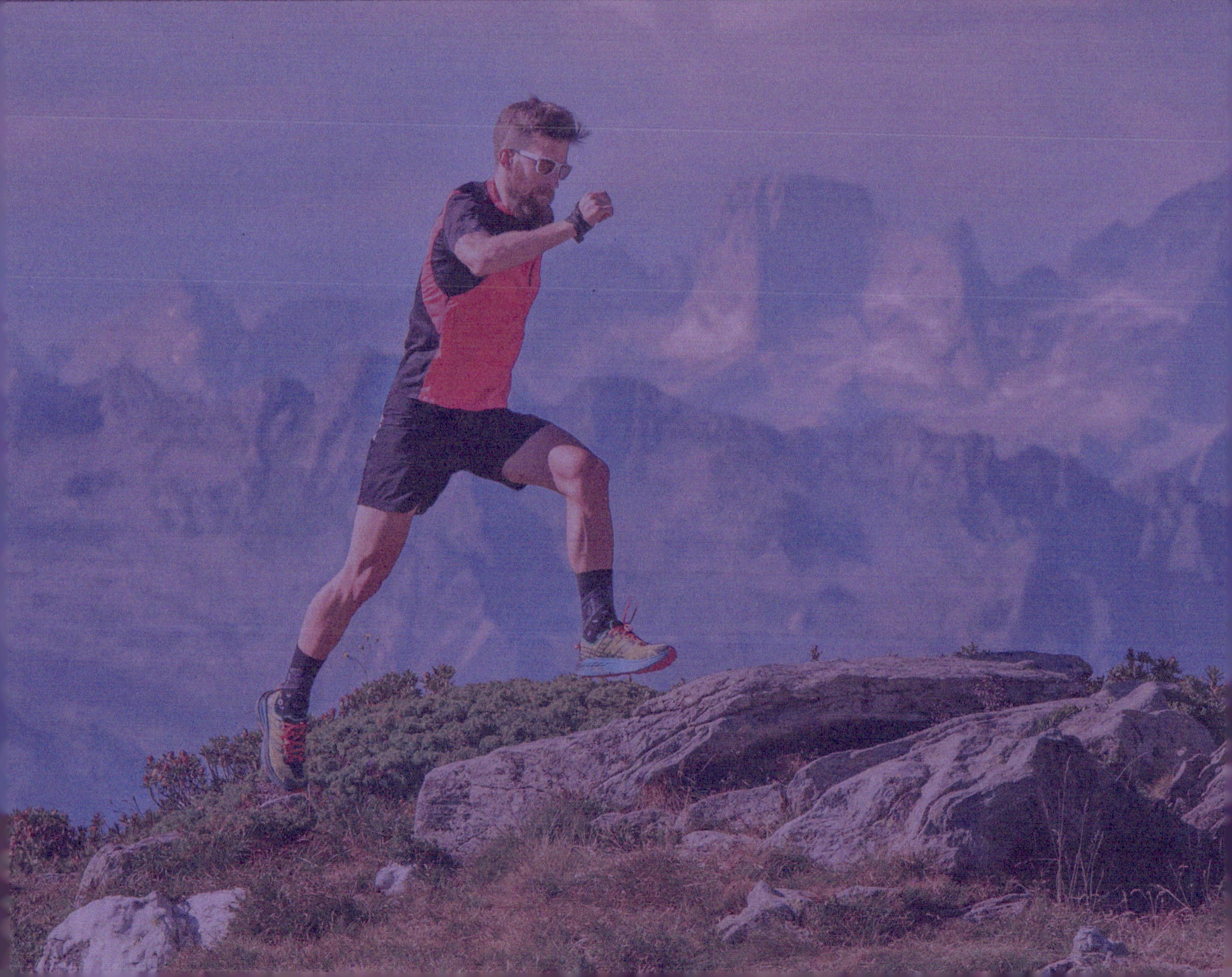

INTRODUCTION

Strong, healthy feet. That's the dream, and with the help of this book, your reality! There's some real homework ahead, but if you're up for the challenge, you'll be rewarded with better balance, a stronger grip on the ground, and a rock-solid foundation for walking, running, or whatever you're into.

As a Canadian Certified Pedorthist with a PhD in Health and Rehabilitation Science, a background in sports medicine and orthopedics, and eighteen years' experience helping tens of thousands of patients find their best footing to aid in injury recovery and prevention, I can tell you that one of the keys to lasting recovery and prevention of future injury is to get strong. How, you ask? The answers to this question are complicated in some ways, and yet devilishly simple in others.

Don't worry! I'm here to help you navigate through our step-by-step approach and have some fun along the way.

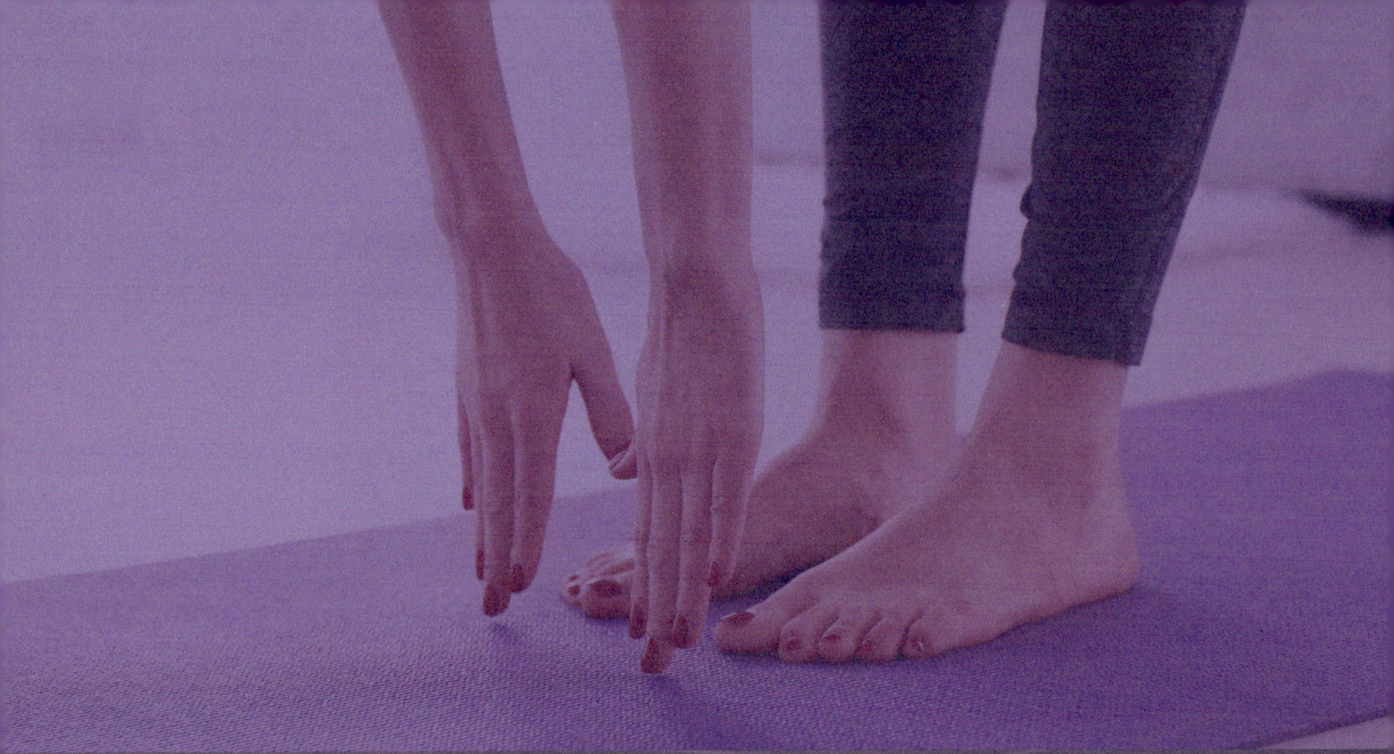

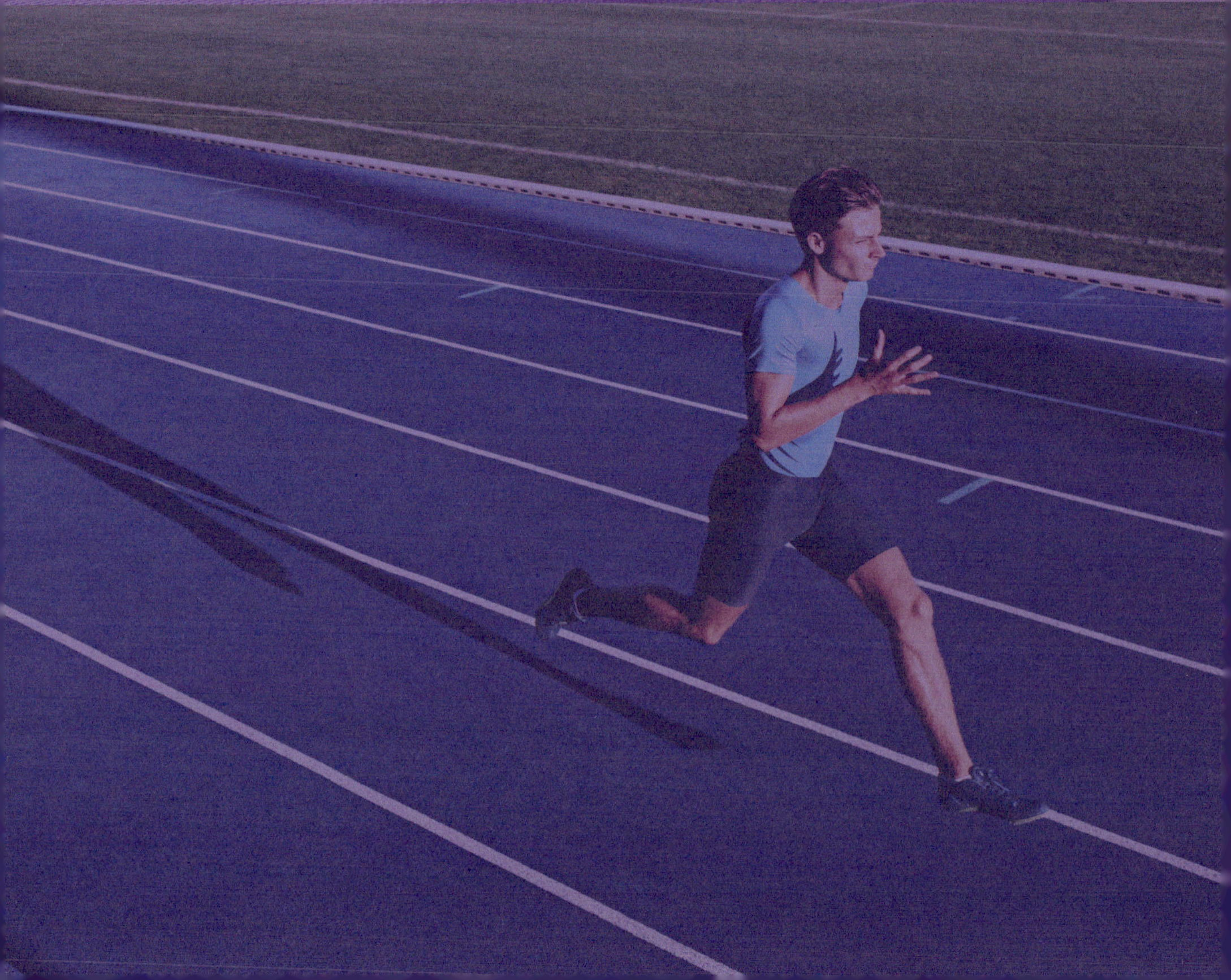

CHAPTER ONE

WHY STRENGTHEN YOUR FEET?

Reducing your risk of injury is the best reason to follow the advice on the coming pages. It's important to remember that while most injuries have just a few causes, they have a lot of solutions. Unfortunately, there's a tendency to think that the latest fad in footwear (either minimalist or maximalist) is the solution to every injury risk factor. Take barefoot running, for instance. Is going barefoot the best option? Should we run "like our ancestors did"? It's just not that simple. For some of us, getting out for a walk around the block is a major achievement. Some can go from couch to marathon barefoot with no problems, while for others trying to train barefoot is downright dangerous. The real question is, what is the best solution *for YOU*? Do you have a history of not getting injured that often? If so, you might be able to do more than the average person. Or, are you someone who suffers from osteoarthritis and has a hard time being active? If so, the approach you need to take may be completely different from the next person / your friend / Usain Bolt.

How can you train effectively, keep practicing your favorite sport, and avoid injury? How do you make sense of all the conflicting information? Most importantly, how do you keep your feet and your body operating at their peak, with full mobility? (As I'll explain later in this book, there's an important difference between just being flexible and being truly mobile.) Why can some people go from sitting on the couch to running a half-marathon with no pain, despite doing it all wrong (at least according to conventional wisdom). Others follow the best advice from world experts and still get injured.

We all have an innate desire for one-phrase answers, simple solutions to complex questions. Spoiler alert: I'm a foot specialist with a PhD, and I still don't know all the answers. Neither do the many "experts," but I can tell you what I do know. The barefoot people will tell you going barefoot is best, while the foot specialists and doctors will have a variety of opinions, and people in shoe stores will pitch in with their advice. What is "right" for a 34-year-old post-partum mom with recent foot changes, a 60-year-old man with knee osteoarthritis who wants to run, and a 22-year-old uninjured college student will be vastly different.

Injury Answers

Let's start with the complicated question of why humans experience injuries differently. Why do some people never seem to get hurt or have only fast-healing minor injuries, while others do similar activities and always get injured? Aren't we all humans who can reach beyond our natural potential and be the machines we were destined to be? I'd argue that such a fate isn't for everyone. The history of foot injury gives us some clues.

Back in the 1950s, the popular theory was that your foot functioned best when it was in its most "neutral" position. You've probably already heard this, because all kinds of foot orthotics, athletic shoes, and exercise forums have been touting the word neutral for decades. It was a convenient theory, because it's both simple to understand and to explain. Trainers, podiatrists, shoe salespeople, and everyone else would say, "See your low arch? That's the reason you have this injury. Let's fix that." As practitioners, we hung our hat on it.

The problem? While it was a convenient theory, it had never been empirically validated. We just grabbed it and went with it, as it was the best information we had at the time. Fast forward to the 1990s, when we learned that the "neutral" theory didn't really work the way we assumed. Oops.

To understand what's wrong with the neutral theory, take a look at the pictures below.

This is the type of thing I see every day. The person in Image 1 *(Image 1)* is what we'd call a classic "over-pronator." Why would that person need orthotics? Just look at that arch! Of course it needs help! (So said every orthotic salesperson, ever.) But in fact, this person is an Ironman triathlete with little to no injury history.

Now look at the next picture *(Image 2)*. Here's the classic "neutral" foot. Look at the beautiful arch. Not too high, not too low—the pinnacle of the normal distribution of feet. But this person is a patient who, despite our multidisciplinary team's best efforts, can't run a 5K without experiencing severe symptoms of plantar fasciitis.

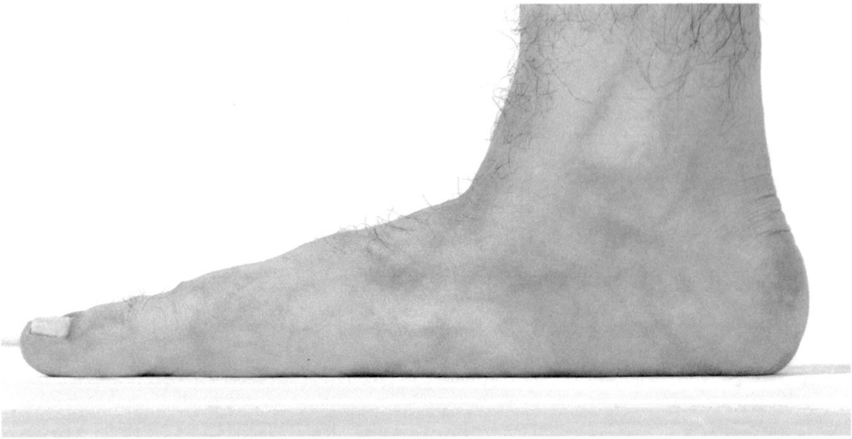

Image 1

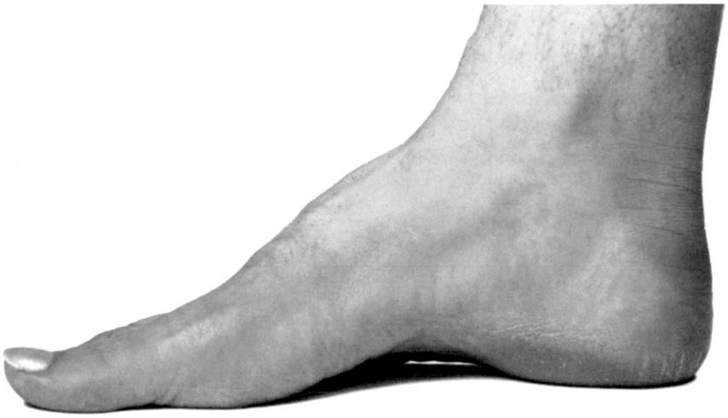

Image 2

Why, you ask? That's the billion-dollar question! (Really: A billion dollar industry was born out of this.) When I lecture to medical, physical therapy, or pedorthic students, I always ask, "How do orthotics and shoes work?" After they give me a blank stare filled with panic, they usually answer with the traditional ideas about better alignment, controlling biomechanics, and my favorite, guiding the foot back to neutrality. While none of that is incorrect per se, I give them another answer. I have no clue at all. Cue nervous laughter. While my answer is not entirely true it's a good wake up call at 7:30 a.m. in a lecture or conference hall.

Actually, no one *really* knows the true mechanism behind how orthotics and footwear work. If anyone claims to know how all this stuff works, run away screaming. Especially the on-line 'Gurus' who tell you it's all coming from your hips or that it's only a foot problem. While the hips and feet are connected, rarely is it ONLY the issue of one or the other, but often it's both together. Dysfunction in one area can and often will show up in another.

Since the 1990s, when we learned that neutrality didn't really work, researchers have gone to work on the question of foot function and how orthotics may influence injury. In the following years, eight competing theories have emerged. None has yet proven to be 'the one.'

Until very recently, traditional 3D motion analysis wasn't able to provide a good solution either. The human foot has 26 bones, 33 joints, and more than a hundred muscles, tendons, and ligaments, all connected in multiple articulations. On top of that complexity, individuals vary hugely in the structure of their feet.

The equipment we used to understand how everything works together just wasn't sensitive enough to give definitive answers. Recent research using fluoroscopy (a moving X-ray) is poised to help provide better answers, but we still have a long way to go.

To see the foot move under fluoroscopy, visit stuffaboutfeet.com

Soft Tissue Stress Theory

My favorite theory and, in my humble opinion, the most clinically elegant, was proposed in 1995 by Thomas G. McPoil, PhD, PT, ATC and Gary C. Hunt, MA, PT, OCS. They call it "soft tissue stress theory," which basically states that injuries are caused by pathological stresses in soft tissues (muscles, tendons, ligaments) in the body. The levels of stress any single soft tissue can handle vary enormously from person to person and from tissue to tissue. Some people have huge zones (more on this in a bit), with a large area of resilient soft tissue that can be extensively stressed yet seldom reach a point from which it can't recover. These people are the lucky ones, like our Ironman competitor (Yay genetics!).

Others just naturally have a smaller or very limited tolerance to soft tissue stress. They will start down the road to injury quickly and take longer to recover when they do get injured.

Variability is what makes us human. We need to know, understand, and own our variability if we wish to overcome it.

Steps Forward from Injury

The zone of healthy soft tissue stress is different for each person. That means we're all on a spectrum of injury and performance potential. On one end of the spectrum are the people who rarely get injured despite doing it all "wrong". Poor sleep, poor nutrition, old or worn-out shoes, and too much, too soon change in activity doesn't seem to bother them. These are the gifted ones—or the genetic outliers. They're the unicorns who do well no matter what they do. (Really, we could just sell them the boxes the shoes came in, coin the term 'box running,' and start the next craze.) In my experience, though, they're the exception, not the rule.

On the opposite end of the spectrum are the people who are often injured, despite following expert advice and doing everything "right." If we represent this data as a bell curve, 70% of us would fall somewhere in the middle. The real question you must answer for yourself is where you are on the curve? Are you in the middle, or do you skew to one of the ends?

Each of us is on a spectrum of athletic potential. All the talk about reaching "more potential than you ever thought possible" is, well, B.S. when comparing person to person. Some of us can never reach that kind of performance, and it's downright dangerous to suggest otherwise, while others go on to do superhuman things. Perhaps you can reach more performance potential, for you, based on your situation and your willingness to try, but not when compared to another human / athlete / anomaly.

In today's world, the strongest aren't the only ones to survive. If a group of us are running from an angry bear, I don't have to outrun the bear for my genes to make it through to the next generation. I just have to outrun you. I don't have to be the fastest; I just need to make sure not to be the slowest. Now, there's nothing wrong with being near the back of the pack—it's fine, and completely normal for some of us. While others gallop like gazelles at the font of the pack, effortlessly. Let's remember this when we visualize the spectrum of human potential. Not all of us were designed to be the physically fittest, yet here we are.

Take yours truly for example. I was already riddled with a brutal type of hip arthritis in my teens, so my ability to run is next to zero (I don't even run to catch a plane!). Due to this, my ability to reach my maximum athletic potential is severely limited. I know and accept this and work hard to make sure I'm as healthy as possible anyway. All of this is to remind us that among humans there is a considerable amount of variability. We need to take that variability into account when we decide how to keep healthy.

This brings me back to the idea that there could be just one theory or just one answer to healing our injuries. If the only tool in your box is a hammer, everything starts to look like a nail.

Just as we should embrace our variability as humans, we should embrace variability in our thinking and solutions when it comes to injury treatment and prevention, whether we are practitioners or patients.

It's time to stop following the one-size-fits-all theories: clinical guru worship; barefoot is better than shod; forefoot is better than heel striking; and pronators always need orthotics. Simplistic answers like these to complex questions can get us into trouble. They lead us down the path where we say, "Barefoot is best for me, and therefore it must be best for you." A logical fallacy.

As a practitioner, I want to produce different, tailored solutions to maximize individual injury prevention, injury recovery, and performance. I want to use a mix of all the tools at my disposal to take your variability and injury history into account. Footwear, orthotics, braces, mobility, strength, and every other approach I know, including diet, sleep, recovery, etc. should be mixed to get the best possible answer for *you*.

CHAPTER TWO

ARCHES AND HOW THEY MOVE

Do you have "normal arches"?

YES! Your feet are NORMAL–They are normal *FOR YOU*.

The way your arch is put together is the sum of your genetics, influenced by injury, pathology, and strength. It's what happens as your arch moves that is considered important, and what researchers have been focused on studying.

The main movements:

Pronation: The feet are rolling TOWARD the midline of the body and are often associated with lower arches

Supination: The feet are rolling AWAY from the midline of the body and are often associated with higher arches

Through the acts to pronation and supination, the arch of your foot transfers your body weight from your heel to your toes when you take a step. Here's where normal variability can easily be seen. Some people naturally have low arches—the height of the arch is below a set average, based on some normal distribution research. Some people have arches so low that they're basically nonexistent—they have flat feet. Lower arched feet, generally, are flexible.

Others have naturally high arches—the height of the arch is above the set average. Most people fall in the middle, with arches that are in between low and high. While knowing your arch type is important for selecting footwear (I'll explain more about this later on), does it affect your risk of injury? Maybe—and maybe not.

If you have a really high-arched foot, however, it is typically very rigid. It doesn't absorb shock very well, which is a necessary function of the foot, and you may wind up with more shock-related injuries as a result.

If you have a normal arch, then your foot doesn't pronate a lot, nor does it supinate a lot. It just moves a little bit in each direction, which is fine.

In all cases of feet, there are exceptions to each type. Deformity such as club feet, Charcot feet etc. may be acquired through genetics, or changes in structure can be the result of injury, medical condition, or dysfunction. This can lead to excessive stiffness or hypermobility in any joint. Sometimes we see flat feet that are stiff and immobile, and in others it's high arches that are highly flexible.

Running magazines, books, and internet are full of articles about how pronation is bad for you. That's not really the whole story. Pronation is the normal movement for most people who have normal to low-arched feet, because it helps to reduce load when you walk or run. Pronation can put more strain on your foot and leg, but remember, having a super-low-arched foot doesn't necessarily cause a problem. Remember the pain free ironman? That might be you. Or perhaps people tell you that your arches are "normal" but you still have pain. What we've been getting at here is that everyone is their own normal.

My course of action for people with flat feet isn't to give them orthotics as a first-line treatment, it's to get them into the right footwear, shoes that complement their individual mechanics and history of pain and injury (if there is any). Additionally, we recommend strength and mobility for the feet and lower legs.

A lot of research has tried to show that a low-arched foot increases the risk of injury or even causes injury. Intuitively, we look at flat or very low-arched feet and say, "Oh, my gosh, look at those things! Of course they're going to cause problems!" That link still hasn't been conclusively established because there are lots of people with low-arched feet who don't get injured. Some studies do show a correlation between low arches and injury, but correlation doesn't mean causation. What we can say, based on the research, is that if you have both low arches and an injury like plantar fasciitis (PF), your low arches may or may not have caused your plantar fasciitis, but they can explain why you're not getting better.

Additionally, some evidence supports the idea that to reduce the likelihood of injury, runners with flat feet should choose footwear that better stabilizes their feet, in addition to strength and mobility.

When we look at the opposite situation, a higher-arched foot, we see a foot that's inflexible, immobile, doesn't absorb shock very well, and doesn't adapt to changes in surface easily. Research estimates that up to 60% of people with high-arched feet experience chronic foot pain. People with high arches are more likely to develop plantar fasciitis and other injuries under the ball of the foot. We can actually take preventative measures with orthotics and footwear for this condition. These techniques can reduce foot pain up to 75%. Speaking with a qualified pedorthist, chiropodist, or podiatrist is your best bet here.

The height of your arch is simply the way you were made. I like to think about people on a continuum, because it elegantly answers the following clinical question: How can some feet be so low-arched that they touch the ground like a pancake but they can run marathons without pain? And how can people who have relatively small deviations from "normal biomechanics" suffer from a ton of pain and problems?

And we haven't even begun to add in other risk factors that may affect your injury potential such as body weight (being over / underweight), genetic predisposition to tendon-related injury, reduced range of motion, how previous injury may affect the function of ligaments, quality of diet and sleep, and the list goes on.

This is where soft tissue stress theory comes into the picture. It's why someone with a so called normal-looking foot can be plagued with problems and pain. Your foot has so many bones, tendons, ligaments, and muscles that it's surprising more doesn't go wrong. The individual variability of how all these elements interact is huge. There are 26 bones in the foot, and the way those bones touch each other and articulate with one another is different for everybody. Some people just have larger joint ranges of motion, while some people just have smaller ones. Some people have no range of motion at all—those foot bones are fused together. Another good reason why trying to fit everyone to one answer—flat shoes are best, for example—doesn't work. Even strength, yes the topic of this book, for some individuals with neurologic disorders, can *negatively* affect them and make them *weaker.*

What Kind of Arch Do You Have?

To help arm you with better knowledge of your foot type, you can do a very simple test at home called the 'wet foot test' or 'the paper test.' This test is credited to Colonel R. I. Harris and Major T. Beath, who used the test on Canadian soldiers to evaluate issues related to their feet. To do the test yourself, open out a brown paper bag or lay some newspaper on the floor. Tape the paper to the floor. Remove your shoes and socks and lightly wet the soles of your feet. Walk across the paper. You'll leave a wet footprint. If you compare the outline to the ones in the diagram below, you can see if you have a high, medium, or low arch. *(Image 3 on next page)*

Based on what you now know about your arch, you can choose the right type of athletic shoe for your foot or have a place to start with respect to strength. To be more precise, you can avoid buying the wrong type of shoe. Running shoe technology has advanced quite a bit over the years, but runners still get injured in their shoes. Evidence shows that getting a shoe that's wrong for your foot type may cause pain. There certainly is not "one best" shoe for everyone, but based on mechanics, there are certainly wrong ones. How can I avoid getting the wrong shoes you ask?

Let's say you have a really high arch and spend more time on the outside of your foot when you run. If you get a shoe that's

THE WET TEST

After dipping your foot in water, step onto a brown paper bag. See which arch type your imprint most closely resembles.

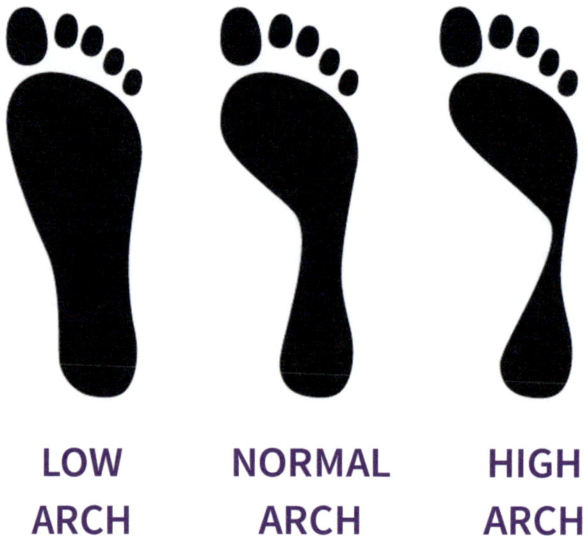

Image 3

designed as an anti-pronation shoe, its job is to try to push you more to the outside of the foot. Since you spend more time on the outside of your foot already, then you might overcorrect yourself and you may get pain on the outside of your ankle or your foot because the shoe is exaggerating what your foot naturally does. If someone who's a supinator—whose foot rolls away from the midline of the body with each stride— gets into an anti-pronator shoe, that would be the incorrect shoe for their foot type. Instead, they want a shoe to either counteract the movement of their foot or complement it. Either will remove some of the strain on the soft tissues. I'll cover more on this in end of Chapter Eight.

A word of caution: Don't get too carried away with the results of the wet foot test, though. Static measures of your feet may not tell the entire story. What happens dynamically as your feet move in the shoes can also affect shoe selection. If you're having foot pain or injuries, I advocate seeing a professional, like a certified pedorthist or podiatrist who can examine your feet and your gait and help you decide what sort of shoe is best for you.

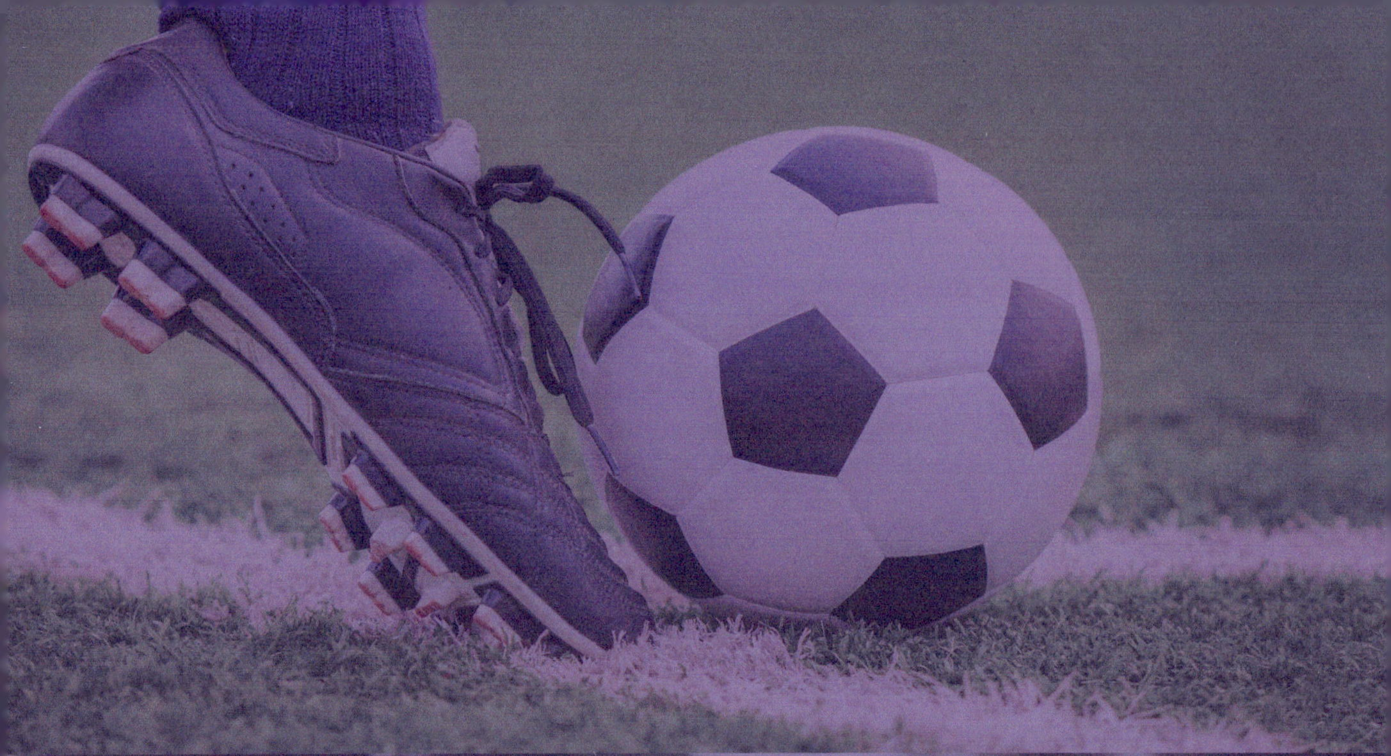

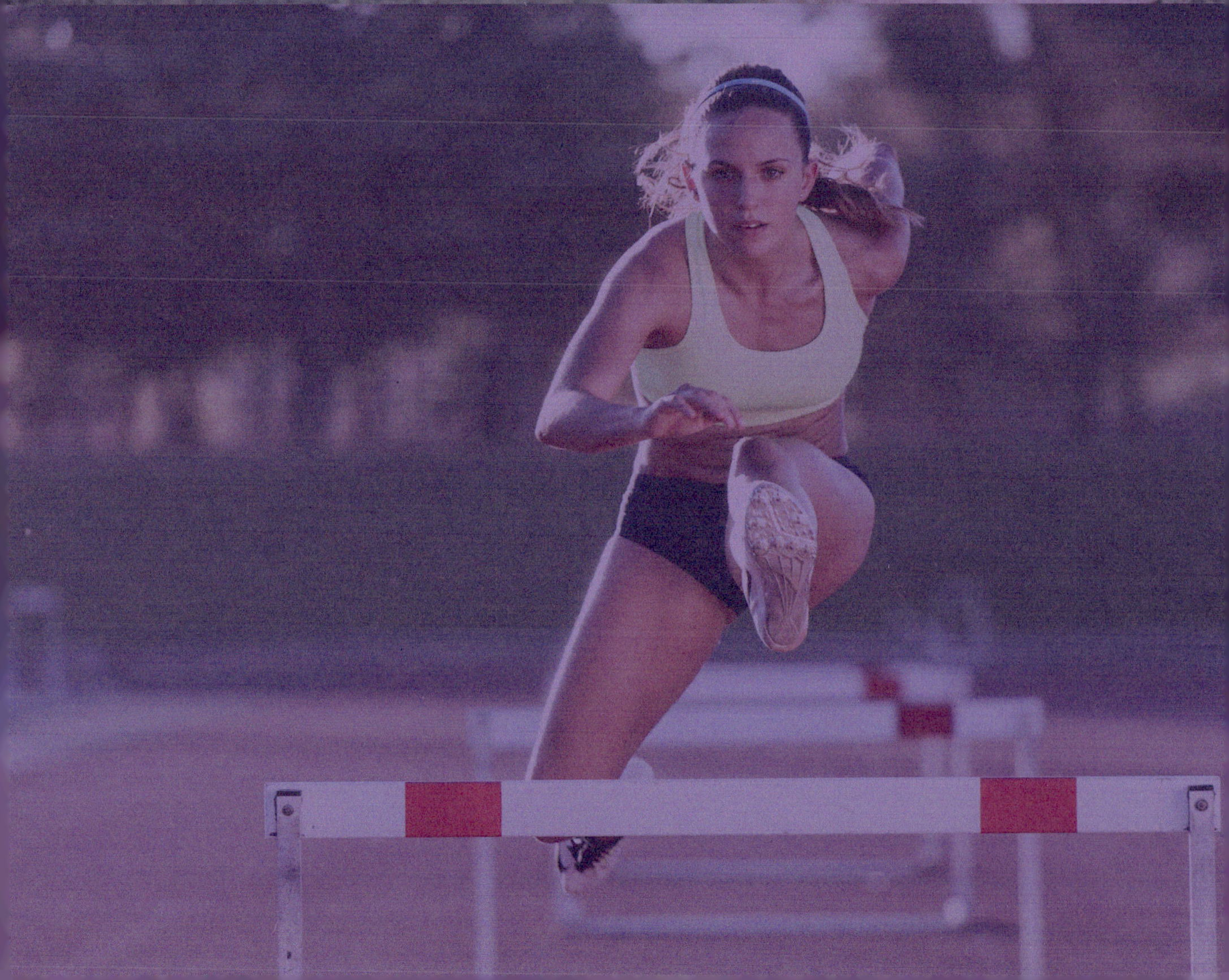

CHAPTER THREE

THE TRUTH ABOUT ORTHOTICS

Custom foot orthotics are commonly used to control abnormal foot mechanics, aid with injury recovery, and provide relief from painful foot pathologies that are either acutely acquired through injury and are not responding well to treatment or are caused by a chronic condition such as arthritis or diabetes. A frequent fear among first-time foot orthotic users, no thanks to scary videos on the internet, is the development of a long-term dependence upon orthotics for comfort and injury-free activity. It's a reasonable concern but, depending on the reason for the orthotics, this may or may not be valid.

Do Orthotics Make Your Feet Stronger or Weaker?

Great question; in fact, it may be *the* question. There are two different schools of thought on this issue.

"WEAKER"

The first, is that orthotics (and / or shoes for that matter) act like a splint or cast, stopping movement and thus creating dependance and / or making your feet weaker. Splinting and casting are used to immobilize a structure while it heals. Orthotics and footwear allow your foot to move while it heals, just in a different way.

Canadian research published in 2020 in the *Journal of Clinical Biomechanics* (I'll refer to this as the "weaker" study from now on) suggested the result for 9 people with flat feet of wearing custom made foot orthotics, was a small reduction in cross sectional area of three foot muscles. Muscle function, however, as tested in this study, did not change during gait tasks. The authors suggested a disuse atrophy or when muscles get smaller from disuse.

Why you ask? The authors suggested the support in the orthotics reduced the need for the muscles in the foot to work, and thus they reduced, slightly, in size *but did not change in their function.*

A common suggestion of "weaker" school of thought is that shoes and orthotics work like casts, immobilizing the foot and making it weaker. I have done research alongside a world renowned group from London Ontario, using biplane fluoroscopy (a moving x-ray) and have proven this is not the case, immobilization does not occur. When we use shoes and orthotics, the foot still moves, just in a different way. Orthotics do not immobilize your foot from moving like a cast does, but rather they modify how the foot moves (slows down actions, limits actions, changes timing of events, compensates for various abnormalities). If you'd like to see videos of the foot in action under a "moving x-ray", just visit, stuffaboutfeet.com.

"STRONGER"

The results of the "weaker" study were in contrast to Korean research published in the *Journal of Back Musculoskeletal Rehabilitation*, which suggested that for 14 people with flat feet, custom foot orthotics increased both the cross sectional area, and increased strength of the foot muscles measured. And that while both groups were stronger after wearing orthotics, the largest gains were made when a strength program was added alongside custom orthotics (I'll call this the "stronger" study).

Why you ask? It could have to do with changing the length tension relationship in the muscles of the flatter feet. The custom orthotics could have allowed the abductor hallicus to work better, and thus get stronger.

WHOM TO BELIEVE?

Based on the rest of this book, by now you're comfortable with the idea that there is no "one thing that works" and that there's only what works for you. Conclusions of the "weaker" study suggested that a strengthening protocol may be effective if prescribed alongside orthoses. There's nothing wrong with that, and it certainly can't hurt.

On the other side, conclusions of the "stronger" study suggested that wearing custom orthoses in a flat foot did make some muscles stronger, but the largest strength gains were had when you combine orthoses and a strength protocol. So at the end of the day, both studies suggest strengthening your feet.

It is important to note that both studies have flaws, and neither can be generalized to the entire public based on only 9 or 14 people. It is also important to know that orthotics can be made hundreds of different ways based on materials, casting, shaping, etc. We can only conclude that the particular devices used in those individual studies was what gave the result, not "all orthotics."

**** BIAS ALERT ****

My professional opinion, and remember I have an orthotic business, is the evidence that exists around the efficacy of orthotics, for people in pain, outweigh the "weaker" study that suggests that while muscle function didn't change, that cross-sectional area was slightly smaller after 12 weeks. Overall, the gains in function, reductions in risk for populations with metabolic disease, and reductions in pain are real, tangible results and a reason why people wear orthotics.

How I Suggest People Consider Orthotic Use

If you have a condition that requires orthotics, and you're concerned about a change, you already have the tools in your hands!

If orthotics are required because of an acute injury, surgery, or pain such as heel pain, forefoot pain or perhaps an injury that is not recovering well, they can typically be used as a tool to aid with recovery. The patient may be able to wean off them once discomfort or inability has been resolved. Remember, we just ***use them as a tool***, not always as a life-long prescription.

If the orthotics are needed because of a systemic disease or long-term pathology / disease such as arthritis, diabetes, or some movement disorders, custom foot orthotics are typically a long-term solution used to improve quality of life and daily comfort.

In both cases, orthotics are used to provide passive support for the foot and thus redistribute pressure and reduce forces, realign joints, reduce (or increase) muscular activity, and reduce soft tissue strain.

But, let's get something clear. Too many people use orthotics. Yup, it's true. My livelihood is based on this stuff, but I'm here to tell you that there is an over-dependence on orthotics. If you don't have chronic pathology (E.g. diabetes, any type of arthritis, Morton's neuroma, thinning fat pads, direct stress from dropped metatarsals, bunions etc.), or any history of injury, and if you have done the hard work to rehab your feet, then you may not need the devices anymore once you recover! I built a business called SoleScience (www.solescience.ca) on this basis of only providing orthoses to those who truly need them, removing them when they no longer need them, and working with patients to strengthen their feet, too. Other "professionals," however, are quick to say on the internet that only .001% of people really need orthotics, and that too is just not true.

This is where things go sideways, in my opinion. Why does it have to be all or nothing? Why is it either orthotics are good or they're a crazy idea that is making the collective feet of the world weak and unhealthy? Oh wait, it's because a rational, individually driven, research based way to think about it doesn't drive clicks / traffic and it's easier to sell controversy than to take a reasonable approach. Remember a common approach to healthcare as a business is 'complicate to profit.'

So how do you avoid getting swept up in this nonsense? When it comes to the professionals you work with, avoid those with an "us against them" or a dualistic "this ONLY works, and that doesn't; MY way is right and their way is wrong" mentality.

If you're a factory worker who experiences some aches and pains at the end of your shift from standing on concrete for eight hours and who doesn't have chronic pain, then wearing orthotics while you work and not any other time could be a reasonable part of a more comprehensive plan. The larger plan may also include strength training to decrease fatigue, proper footwear to address the issues that may or may not arise from steel-toe boots not fitting properly, a mobility plan that addresses range of motion issues, and a host of other whole-individual solutions. A combination of strategies is often needed to keep you feeling great so that on the weekends you can go out and perform in adventure races or keep up with your kids.

Keep your mind open and with the right approach and professionals to help, you can try and find the options that work best for you.

There is excellent research into the efficacy of orthotics as a treatment for people living with osteoarthritis and diabetes (just to name two—there are more, but you'll get the picture). In the US, in 2013-2017 the Centers for Disease Control reported that it was estimated that 9.4% of the population has diabetes, and that 22.7% of the US population have been told by their doctor that they have "some type" of arthritis. Both statistics affected by the fact that 39.8% of the population over the age of 18 are obese. So much for only .001% of the population, huh? This quite literally means that orthotics as a treatment is more than effective for tens of millions of people across the U.S. alone!

While foot orthotics are used as a form of passive support, physical therapy / Kinesiology is commonly used as a form of active support. It serves to improve muscular strength, flexibility, endurance and to aid recovery from various injuries. Sometimes, foot mechanics can be altered due to poor mechanics or weakness higher up the chain. Weak glutes (butt muscles), can cause your knee to drive toward the midline of your body, keeping your foot in a more pronated position. This is only one example of where things can go awry. But again, be wary of the ones telling you that pronation is ONLY caused or altered by one factor (poor hip mechanics for example). Foot care professionals commonly work alongside physiotherapists to improve factors such as balance, lower limb flexibility, and lower limb strength.

Until recently, however, little attention has been given to the muscles inside the foot. Strengthening these muscles may provide a form of internal support, potentially reducing injury. If the foot is more prepared to support the weight of the body and to respond to various daily activities, it seems fairly intuitive that this may result in reduced injury rates and a better environment for injury recovery. Fortunately, there is some recent research to support this notion. Donella et al suggests that when the intrinsic muscles of the foot are fatigued, the arch drops more, which may lead to increased pronation (Donella, 2008). Now, is this particularly a bad thing? We're not sure. Remember, pronation itself is not an excellent predictor of injury. Pronation is, however, a motion that will place more strain on the soft tissues of the foot / ankle, and demand more of the ligaments and tendons that control it. It would stand to reason that with increased resistance to fatigue, through strength, you can remove some of the resultant soft tissue stress. Alleviating stress on the foot by strengthening higher up the kinetic chain would also be a good idea, although no the focus of this book. For more on that, I'd recommend Kelly Starrett's book, *Becoming a Supple Leopard* (I'll touch on this later).

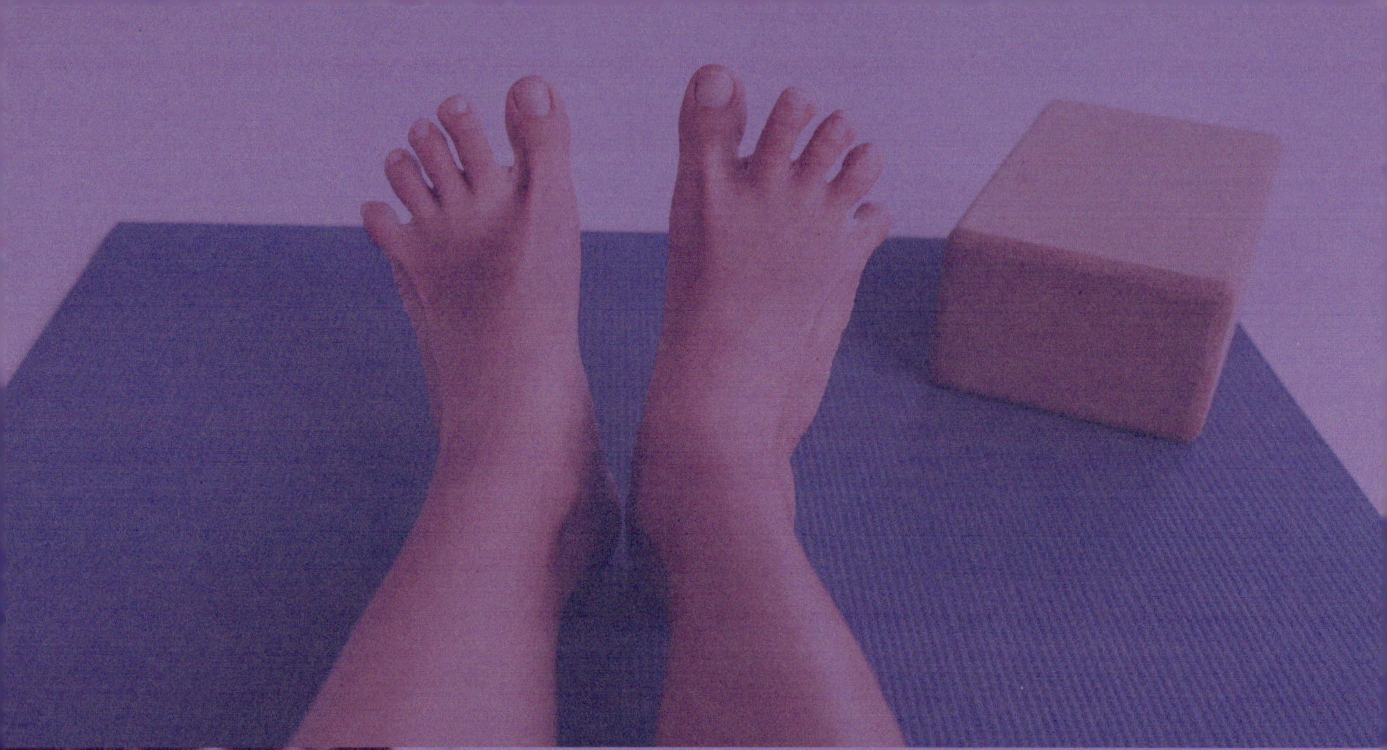

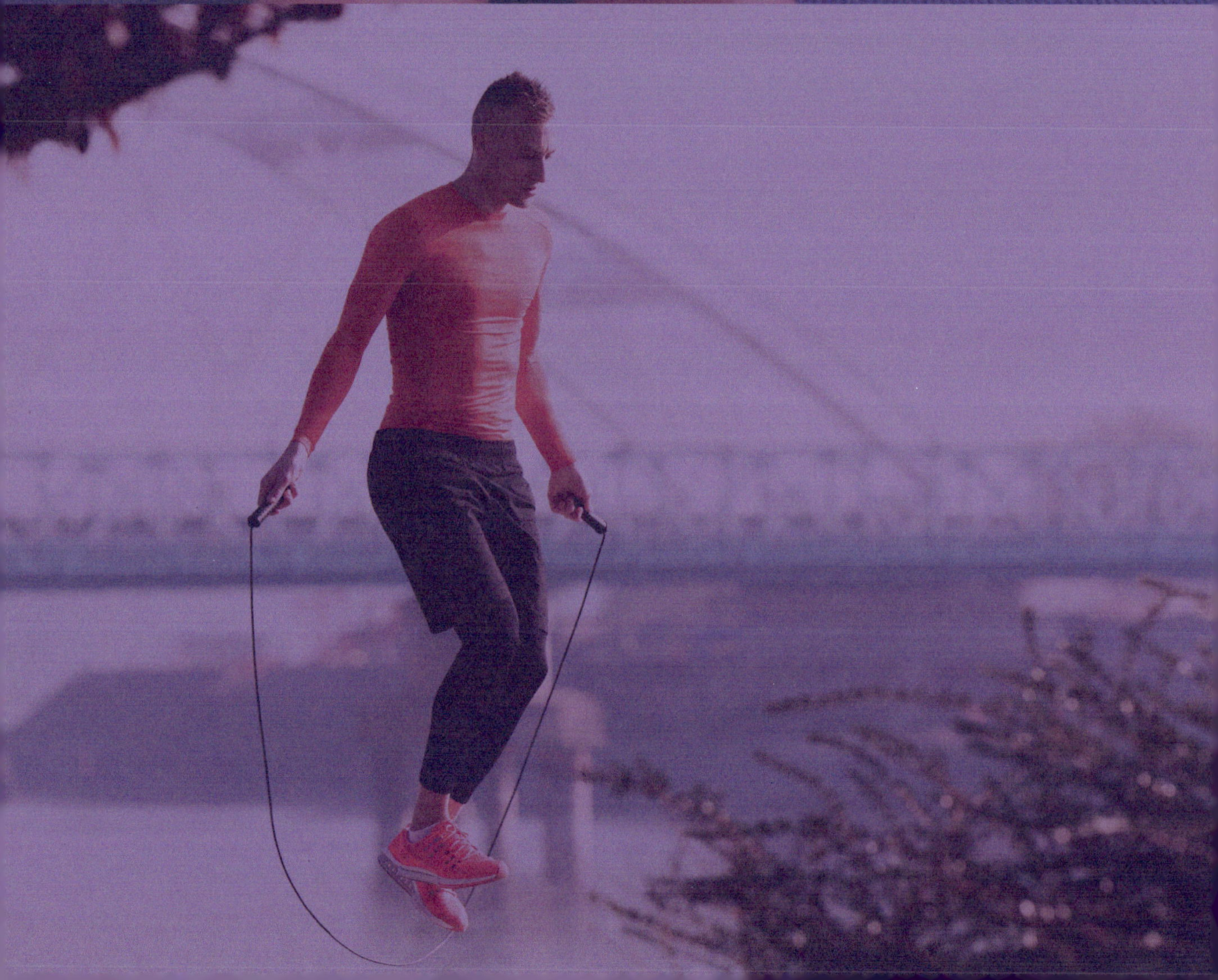

CHAPTER FOUR

FUNCTIONAL ANATOMY & AN EXPERT INTERVIEW

Let's break it down. The bottom of the foot has four distinct layers of muscles, all with important functions. As a whole, this grouping of muscles is used to stabilize the foot—that's why they're called the 'local stabilizer' muscles. Research published in the Journal of Clinical Biomechanics found that the demand for the intrinsic muscles used to stabilize, increased during single leg standing, and when forces acting side to side increased. Or simply put, foot muscles work harder when the need for stability increases, side to side. In the real world, this is particularly important for people who load their foot more often and in different positions, such as the case in any aggressive side to side sport like soccer or basketball, plyometric training or even hiking, where the terrain is often varied. Of course, these are not the only applications, but you get the point. With this in mind, these muscles do not necessarily produce movement of the foot: their role is to support and stabilize the foot while larger muscles in the lower leg generate foot movements. The muscles in the lower limb, also known as 'global mover' muscles, are responsible for movements in all directions.

According to researchers at Harvard Medical School and the University of Delaware, the local stabilizers and global movers are part of a larger system called the 'foot core system.' This system comprises three interacting components: the active subsystem, the passive subsystem, and the neural (nerves) subsystem. The active subsystem is divided into the global mover muscles and the local stabilizer muscles that act together to produce the forces needed to create movement.

The passive subsystem consists of the bones, ligaments, and plantar fascia in the foot and is responsible for giving the foot its shape and providing attachment points for the muscles. The neural subsystem comprises the sensory receptors embedded in the tissues of both the active and passive subsystems. Input from these receptors is used to gain information about the environment and how the body needs to respond to it.

Research indicates that the interaction of these three subsystems is important for the normal functioning of the foot, especially in cases of increased demand, such as running or having an active lifestyle.

But what good is research if you cannot put it into practice? By training the stabilizers, you can improve the function and interaction of the foot core. It is reported that the movement of these muscles not only stabilizes the foot while the muscles in the leg (global movers) contract to produce foot movement, but also that they provide valuable sensory feedback through the sensory receptors in the neural subsystem. This feedback helps maintain the posture and arches of the foot while in use. When the passive movers become fatigued, their ability to provide sensory feedback reduces, and the posture of the foot may be compromised. Increasing the strength and endurance of these muscles with specific exercises has been shown to increase both the activity and size of the important passive stabilizer muscles.

Let's Take a Look at These Muscles

MOVERS:

- flexor hallucis longus / peroneus longus, brevis
- flexor digitorum longus
- tibialis posterior, tibialis anterior

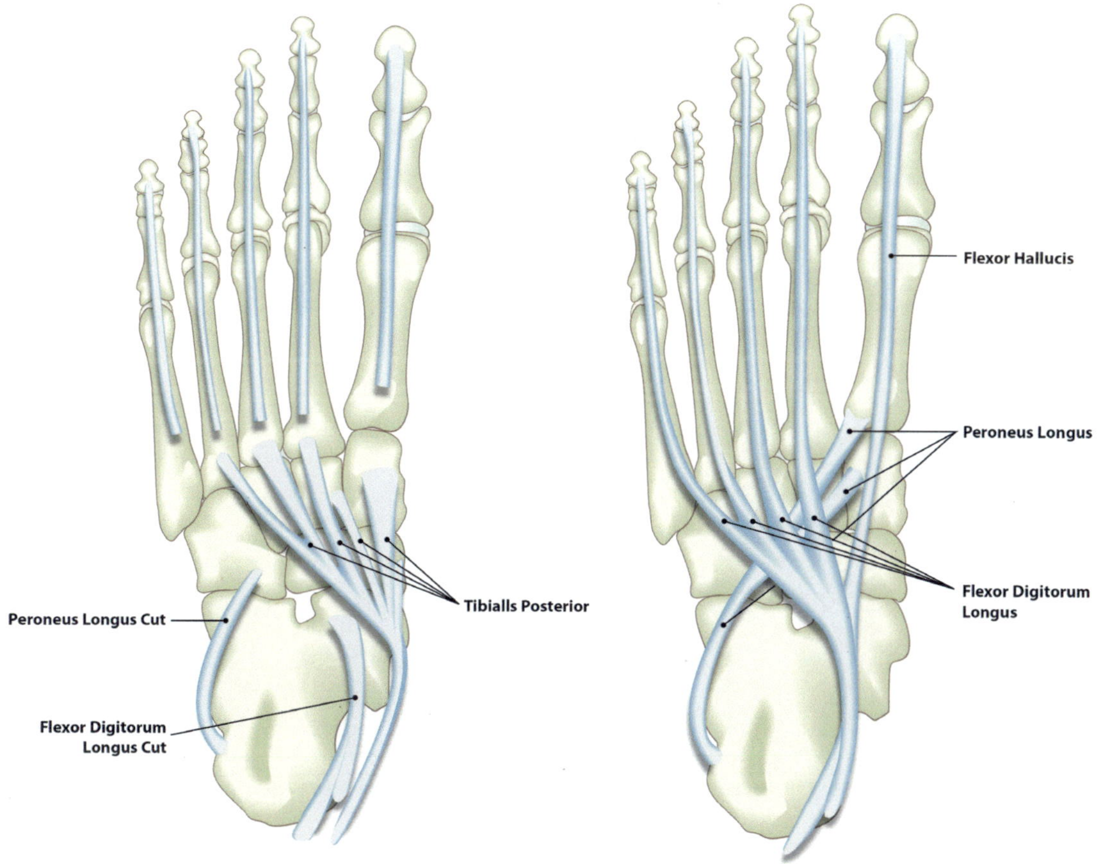

STABILIZERS:

- abductor hallucis
- flexor digitorum brevis / longus
- abductor digiti minimi
- quadratus plantae
- lumbricals

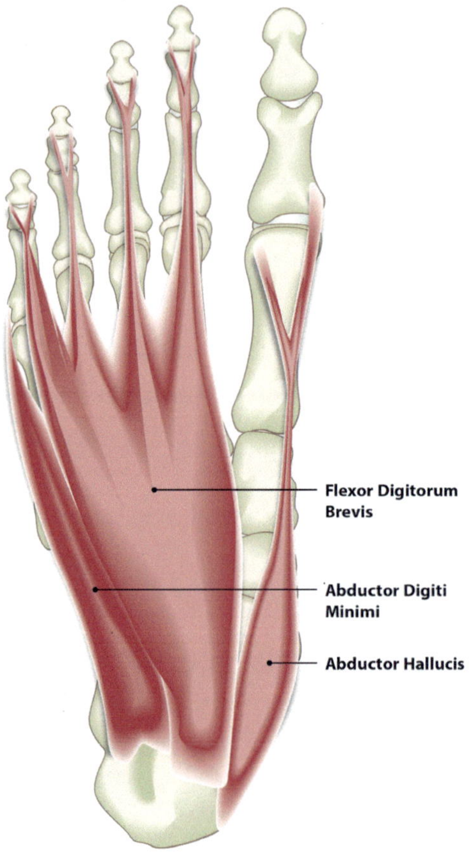

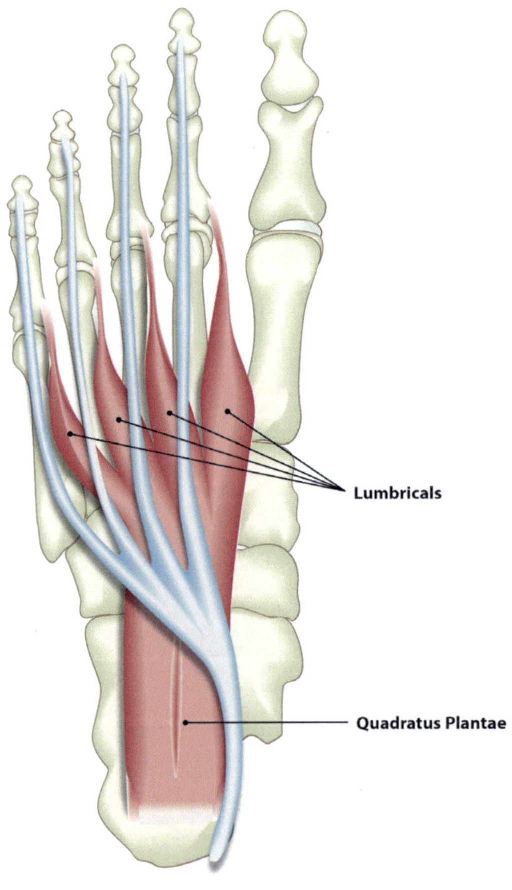

- flexor digiti minimi
- adductor hallucis oblique and transverse heads
- flexor hallucis brevis
- plantar interossei
- dorsal interossei and extensor digitorum brevis

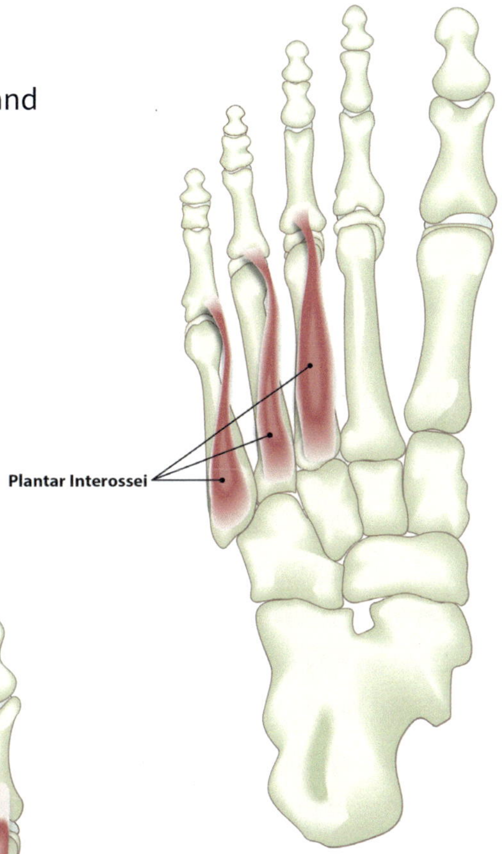

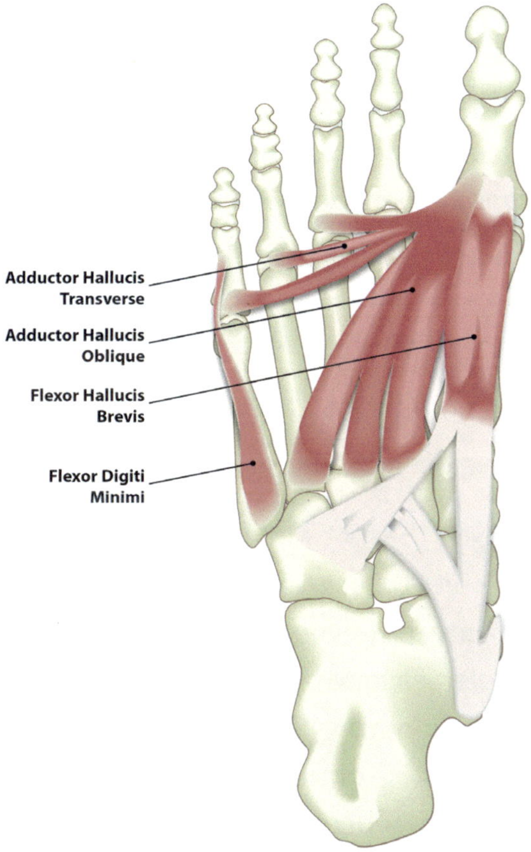

Expert Interview

In one of my other books, *The Plantar Fasciitis Plan*, I had the good fortune of discussing foot strengthening with Dr. Irene S. Davis, PhD, PT, FAPTA, FACSM, FASB, director of the Spaulding National Running Center and the Department of Physical Medicine and Rehabilitation, Harvard Medical School. Dr Davis is leading the charge for foot strength and was one of the authors of the strength paper I referenced above. We talked about how strength in particular helps with cases of plantar fasciitis.

If you've ever had an injury like plantar fasciitis (usually pain on the bottom of your heel when you get up after long periods of rest / sleep) or a foot injury, you can get it again. In that case, it may return with a vengeance. While your first bout of plantar fasciitis may have responded to just six weeks of therapy, your second bout could take as long as two years to heal completely. That's why prevention is critical. Building up your foot strength is a crucial part of preventing a relapse. When the small muscles deep inside your foot are strong, you will feel the effects of fatigue much later in the day. This will help keep your feet feeling great all day long and avoid strain on your plantar fascia.

Dr. Davis shared her thoughts about the role of orthotics and the value of exercise for strengthening the feet. She says,

> "I do think there's a place to support the foot with orthotics in certain situations. I don't think orthotics are the Evil Empire. My overall sense, however, is that they're overused for musculoskeletal injuries. I actually think that in the acute phase, supporting the foot with an over-the-counter orthotic device or taping is a good idea. The foot is just like any other body part. If it's injured, you don't want to have it moving, so you

splint it, let it rest and heal. If someone has severe plantar fasciitis in the acute phase, the last thing you want to do is have them go without support."

I asked Dr. Davis what her advice would be for preventing the recurrence of plantar fasciitis. She replied,

> "Keep the feet strong and flexible. I believe that you have small muscles in your feet that are stabilizers and not prime movers, just as you have muscles in your deep core that act in the same way. To have normal movement of the foot, I think you have to have a very stable foot core, just as you need a very stable lumbar core to prevent back pain. To have a stable, strong foot core, you need to focus on the intrinsic muscles, the ones that originate and insert in the foot. Of the intrinsic foot muscles, the ones to really focus on are the plantar muscles. You've got to do exercises that try to resist the deflection of your arch under load, because that's what strains the plantar fascia and gives it a repetitive load type injury."

So what exercises does Dr. Davis recommend? She says,

> "I think doming [also called arch lift or Janda's short foot] is probably one of the best exercises, because it works all the muscles that are underneath the foot. I recommend getting started with doming and other foot exercises as soon as you can do them without pain. Use your pain as a guide. Pain is your body's way of saying 'you know, this is too much load for me right now.' It's a warning signal, a gift we're given. We use pain as a guide to customize treatment for each patient."

Dr. Davis also observes,

> "You can incorporate doming into your everyday activities, such as while you're standing in line at the grocery store checkout. We teach people how to do active standing, which starts with the foot but also includes some gluteus maximus and lower abdominal activation. It's amazing how different their posture looks when people start to do this. When I work with patients doing physical therapy for plantar fasciitis, we start with doming while sitting, then move on to doming while standing on two feet, then standing on one foot, then doming and hopping on two feet, then doming and hopping on one foot. It's a progression, just like any other exercise program, that moves from static to dynamic to more functional activities. I recommend doing your foot exercises ahead of an activity like running. The exercises activate the foot muscles and make you aware of them right from the start."

We discussed why some people have a second bout of PF. Dr. Davis feels this is because doctors providing treatment fail to emphasize or even think about foot strengthening. She says,

> "We think of the foot as a passive structure, so we don't think about strengthening it. I think one reason we have an epidemic of plantar fasciitis is that we're in supportive shoes all the time. In most cases, people probably don't need all that extra support. We're designed to go barefoot. When we wear minimal shoes without support or go barefoot, we strengthen the foot muscles. I think for treating PF we need to take the simplistic approach. Let the foot do what

> it was designed to do. In therapy, I give every foot a chance to be what it was naturally designed to be. By teaching our patients how to do foot exercises, we're able to wean almost all of them off their orthotics."

We also talked about the benefits of increasing foot strength beyond curing and preventing plantar fasciitis. She told me,

> "You avoid injuries to the foot. The majority of foot problems trace back to weak or imbalanced muscles. Foot exercises can help avoid bunions, stress fractures, and other problems."

(To find out more, please refer to the paper by McKeon et al. 2015, listed in the bibliography.)

Even though this area of research is in its infancy, one research group had this to say regarding intrinsic strengthening: "The absence of evidence does not necessarily indicate evidence of absence in the benefits that isolating the plantar intrinsic muscles offers for outcomes related to lower extremity overuse conditions." Having said that, it's not hard to understand that strengthening your feet is a good thing for your overall foot health! I am always cautious about the people who jump on the bandwagon and say that this type of training is THE ONLY thing one should be doing to resolve a foot and or lower extremity issue. We differ so widely as humans that there are no one shot cures. Frankly, you should avoid those selling the *one thing* to cure everything that ails you.

STRENGTH / MOBILITY + YOUR FEET = THE PLAN

The protocol we recommend works in stages, and each stage builds on previous ones. Like any other plan, adherence to it is where you're going to see progress. We're going to focus on the following steps:

1. **Mobility:** There's little point in getting so strong if you can't execute a proper range of motion. Walk like a duck? We can teach you to work on that.
2. **The intrinsic (deep foot) muscles:** These are the muscles that stabilize your foot and help fend off fatigue.
3. **The extrinsic (surface) muscles:** These are the primary movers of your foot and ankle.
4. **Balance and coordination**
5. **Dynamic stability:** This is where things get fun (and crazy hard).

It's important to note that while each stage builds on another, once you've moved from step one to step two, keep doing all the work of the previous step, too.

CHAPTER FIVE

STEP ONE: MOBILITY

Flexibility vs. Mobility

To avoid injury, you need to have both flexibility and mobility in your feet and ankles. Let's define these two words.

Flexibility: the ability of your muscle(s) to lengthen.

Mobility: your ability to move a joint through its intended full range of motion with strength *in a functional way.*

Flexibility is important for proper joint mobility. To develop flexibility without regard for mobility is asking for trouble, though. It's possible to have great flexibility and poor mobility. Hamstrings can be flexible when testing them, and due to instability somewhere else higher up the chain, for instance with an unstable pelvis or bad posture, be overactive and tighten during gait, affecting the ability to touch one's toes. As we age, our range of motion naturally decreases. You can counteract that natural tendency by staying fit and doing things like yoga that help keep you flexible and your joints mobile. This will really help reduce the likelihood of injury.

One of the most deleterious losses of mobility I see day to day is the loss of range of motion at the ankle. This loss of mobility can lead to decreased stability and increases the loads on both the plantar fascia and the Achilles tendon. Similarly, if your calf muscles aren't sufficiently flexible to allow your leg to move over the top of your foot when you walk, your body compensates for the movement somewhere else. The easiest way to compensate is to pronate your foot (roll it in) or raise your heel prematurely, or some combination thereof. That puts even more strain on your lower extremities.

Your feet can't work properly if you're duck-footed (where your feet rotate externally), so work on fixing that first.

Mobility Exercises to Get the Ankle Moving Better

Do you walk like a duck? Do your feet turn outward when you walk (external rotation)? *(Image 4)*

Can you extend your leg and easily point your toes back toward your shins? *(Image 5)*

This movement is called 'dorsiflexion.' (Pointing your toes down, away from your ankle, is called 'plantarflexion.') If you have a reduction in the dorsiflexion of the ankle, it usually comes from tight calf muscles or some type of restriction in the ankle, such as bone deformity or a build up of scar tissue.

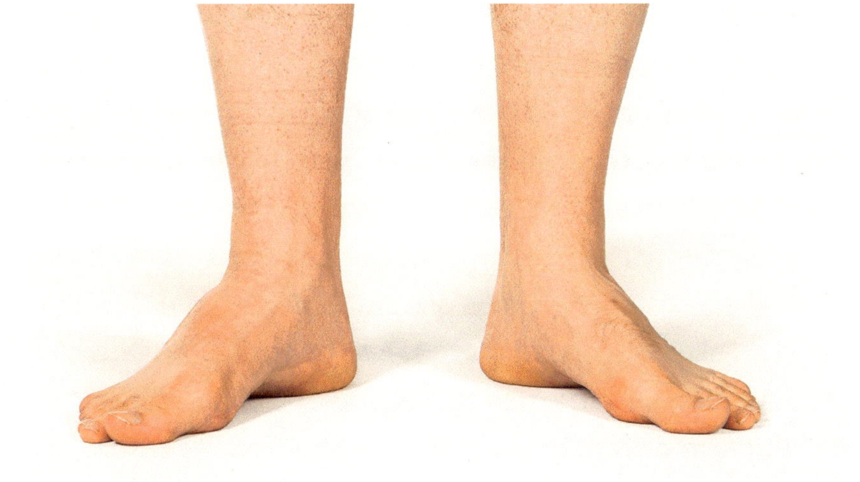

Image 4

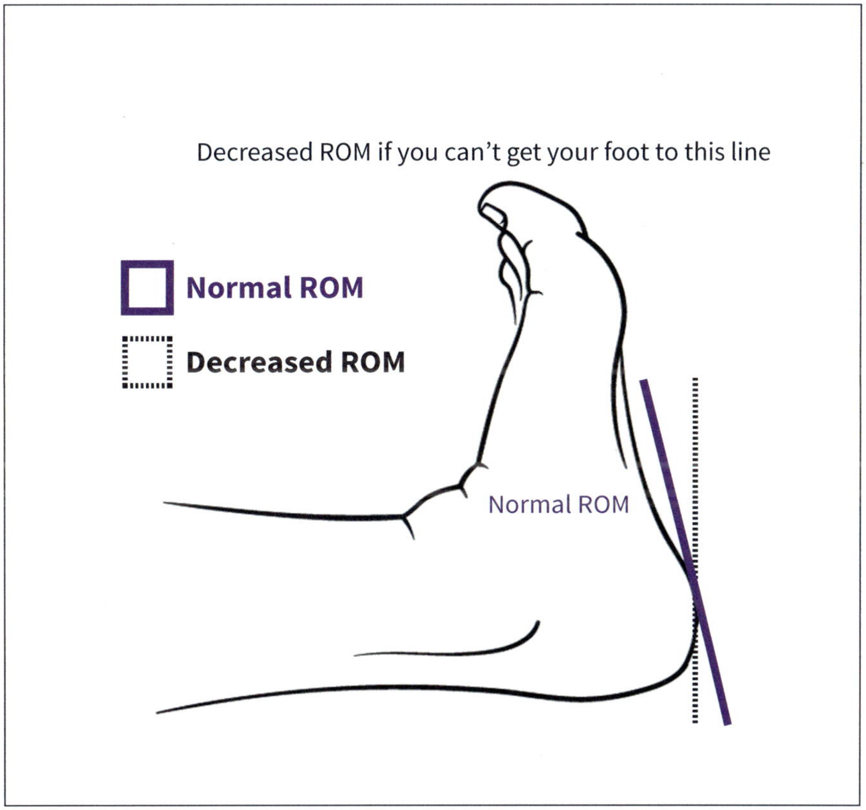

Image 5

Reduced dorsiflexion can be a mechanical determinant in plantar fasciitis (Bolivar et al. 2013). The reason is a little complex. For you to be able to walk, your body must get your leg over the top of your foot. That sounds simple, but if you have biomechanical abnormalities that resist that movement, you have to compensate in some other way. When you have inadequate dorsiflexion, you still have to get your body forward somehow. Your foot is going to make compensations to allow you to do that. One way is to out-toe your foot, which causes you to pronate more. When you out-toe and pronate, you put more strain on the tissues of the lower extremity. Another way to compensate is to lift your heel off the ground sooner than you typically would. Again, that increases strain on your plantar fascia. Some people will do a combination of these. It all leads to more mechanical loading of the plantar fascia and a greater risk of the damage that ultimately causes PF, or other injuries / pain to the feet.

Massage / Rolling / Etc.

Let's start the talk about self-massage or deep tissue release with the calf muscles. The two large superficial muscles at the back of your leg play a major role in shock absorption as you walk / run, help stabilize and balance your leg as you move over your foot and ankle from double to single leg stance, and assist with propulsion as you push off with your toes.

With all the work the calves do, it's no surprise that they are a common source of problems in the lower extremities. If you've ever tried to foam roll your calves, you know how tight and painful they can be!

Tight calf muscles can lead to problems both in the foot and shin, as well as in the knee, hip, and back.

There are two primary muscles in the calf region that we're going to discuss: the gastroc and the soleus. Let's take a look.

The gastroc is the big fleshy muscle at the top of the calf and is the easiest one to spot. The soleus muscle lies just underneath the gastroc, lower down the leg. These muscles share a common insertion with the Achilles tendon, which inserts into the back of your heel and then fans out. The main difference between the two muscles is in how they work. The gastroc crosses the knee joint, while the soleus does not. The gastroc helps you push off with your toes when the knee is *straight*, while the soleus helps you push off while the knee is *bent*.

Self-administered Soft Tissue Release Techniques

What you'll need: a foam roller and a tennis / trigger point ball. If you really feel masochistic, there's a foam roller called a Rumble Roller that has extra-large bumps and really lets you dig into those hard-to-reach spots. It's not for the faint of heart, though, so go slow!

WHAT WE'RE WORKING ON:

- Elongation / lengthening with the foam roller
- Cross friction with the tennis ball
- Sustained pressure / trigger point release with the tennis ball

WHERE WE'RE FOCUSING:

- **The gastroc (the big calf muscle that you see when you flex).** Since both the gastroc and soleus start around this area, it can be full of knots and tender spots. Both foam rolling with an emphasis on the outside of the leg and a hard ball in the same area, or even your thumbs to apply pressure, will work. It's like a choose-your-own-adventure (of torture!) game. Press deep and hold while pointing your foot as far down as it will go, then raise it as far back toward your shin as it will go. Try this for one to four minutes in the beginning. *(Image 6)*

- **The musculo-tendinous juncture (where gastroc and soleus become the Achilles tendon).** Just go easy on this area. It also has the least blood flow, so you don't want to overdo it.
- **The deep posterior compartment.** We didn't really touch too much on the muscles in this compartment, but they are important ones, as it can be a major source of foot and shin pain. While it's deeper in the leg than the larger gastroc / soleus muscles, you can find it like this:

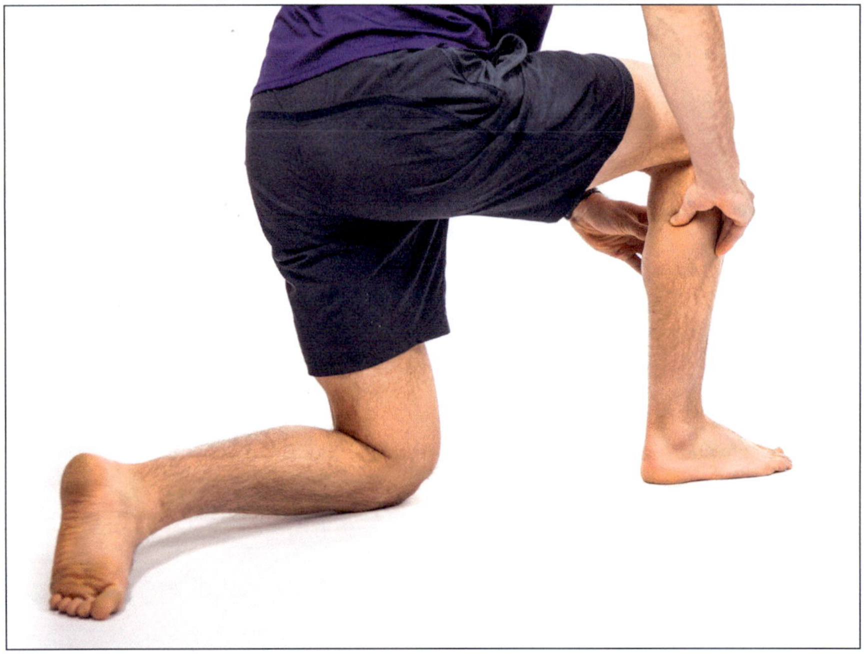

Image 6

1. Place your thumbs on the middle of the tibia, then slide the thumbs back until you're on the muscle. *(Image 7)*
2. Supinate your foot—move it to the inside.

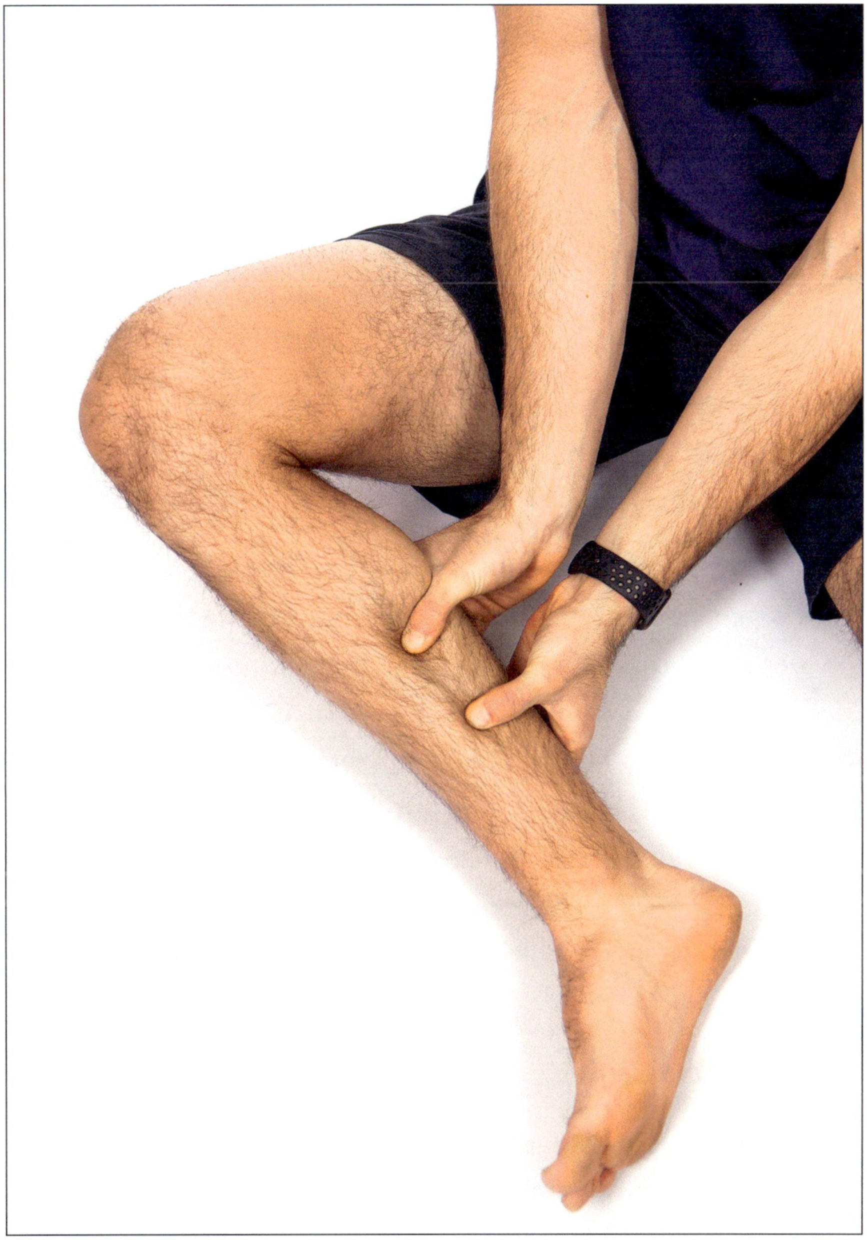

Image 7

3. You will feel the tib post move under your thumbs.

4. Apply a deep pressure with your thumbs / ball.

5. Move around the area about 12-14 cm.

6. Go slow, as the tib post can be very sore and tender to the touch.

Remember to drink lots water after deep tissue sessions to ensure recovery. Repeat the above every one to three days (depending on how sore you are).

EXERCISE:

Ankle mobilization

If your ankle needs some work to help get the range of motion going again, here is a simple mobilization exercise that places the toes up on the wall, essentially making it more of a mobility challenge, and stretching your ankle and posterior calf muscles. The dynamic part of this mobilization technique is what brings real, measurable change to the muscles you're targeting in the calves. Remember, those are huge muscles designed to handle literally tons of load, and you need a better method of change than simple static stretching.

With this technique, you can work on moving the ankle straight, inward, and outward:

1. Stand around 2 feet away from the wall. Position the ball of your foot up on the wall in front of you, heel to the ground. Remember to keep your knee straight. *(Image 8)*

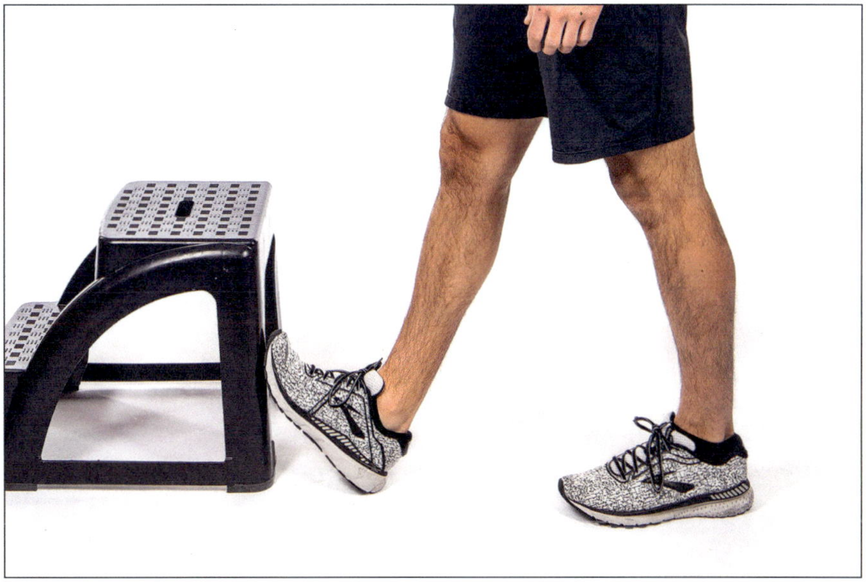

Image 8

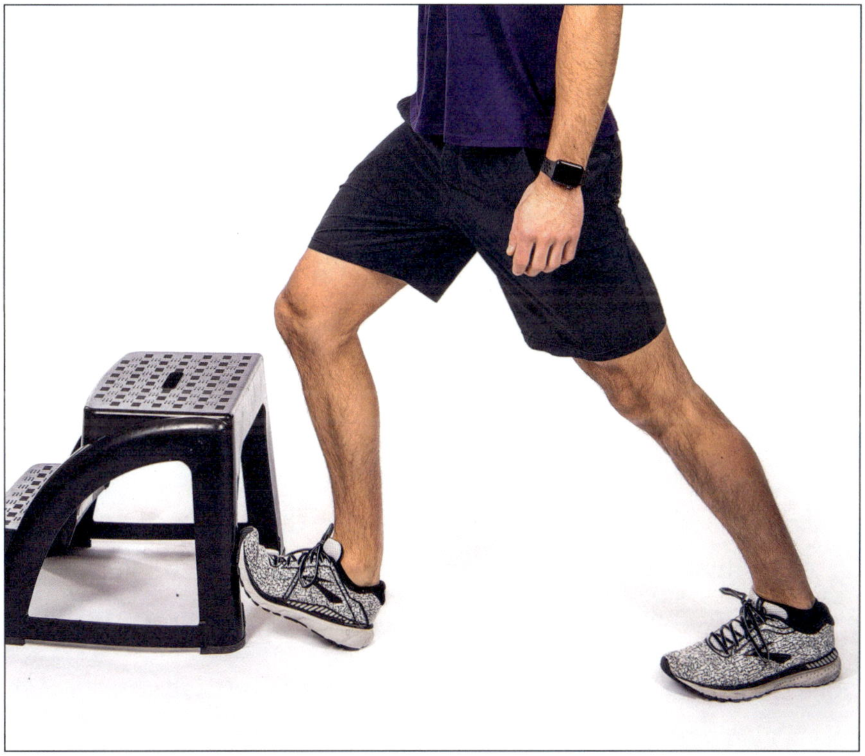

Image 9

2. Keeping your foot in a neutral position, knee straight and body tall, drive your weight straight from your hips towards the wall. *(Image 9)*

3. Try and find different areas of tightness by bending the knee, and moving the knee in internal and external rotation.

(Visit stuffaboutfeet.com to see this technique in action.)

Foam Rolling

Are your calves REALLY sore? I mean, if someone touches them or presses them, do you want to scream? This is what happens when your calves are tender from extreme tightness. Self-soft tissue release might be overly aggressive in this case, so foam rolling might be a good place to start. Why this is important is that reductions in ankle range of motion from tight / sore calves can be a major risk factor for foot and lower leg injury. Combine that with other risks like being overweight, and the compensations needed by your body are not good for your feet. That's why we've spent the time here to get things moving again. Another interesting note is travel. It is always surprising to me how many people come back after a trip with lots of uphill walking, with new foot pain and tight calves. *(Image 10)*

1. Sit with the roller just in front of your knee.

2. With light pressure on both legs, roll to the heel and back again. As this becomes easier and less painful, you can increase the intensity of the roll by placing one leg over the other.

Once that's easy too, revisit the self-soft tissue release. *(Image 11)* This is also a good place to start with a massage therapist / physio who can help ease you into it too, if you're overly tight.

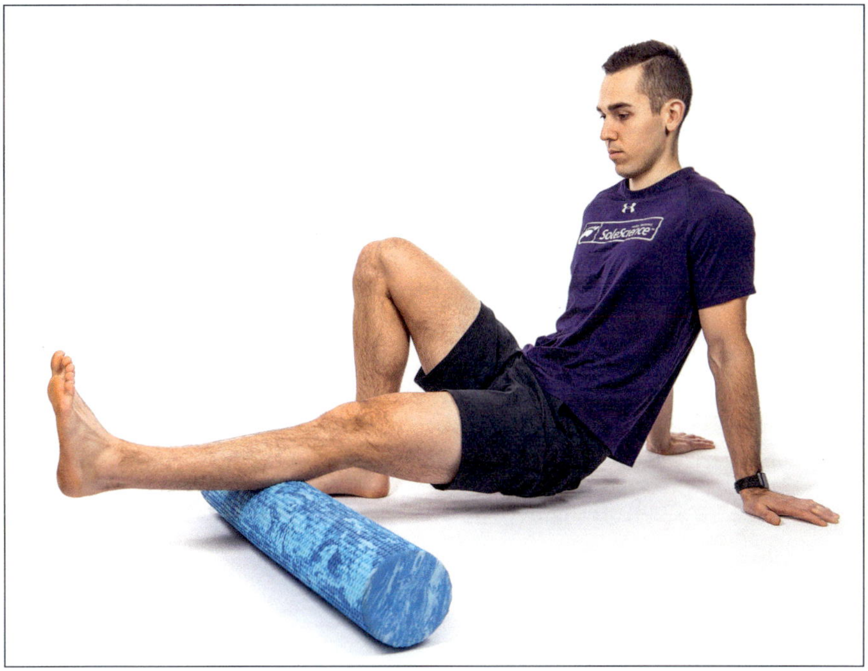

Image 10

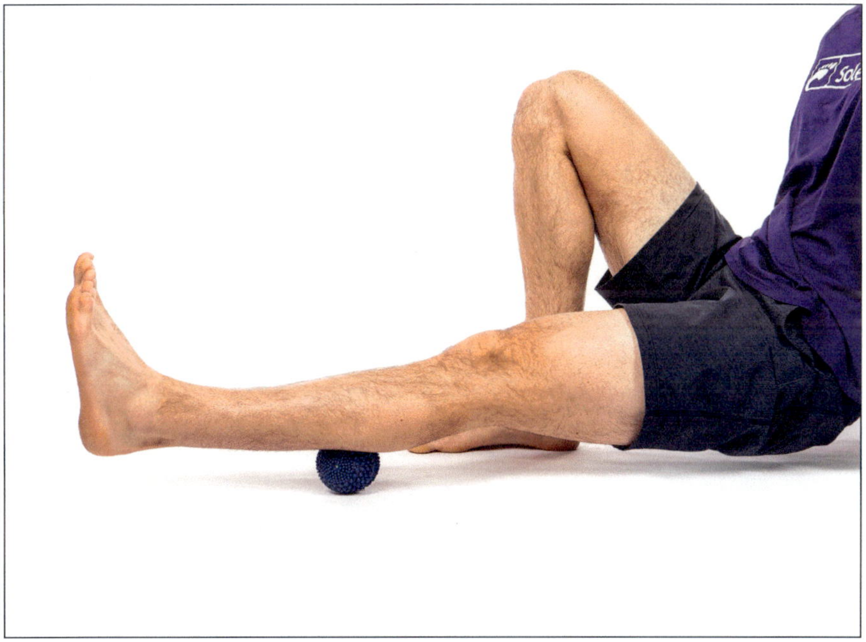

Image 11

EXERCISE:

Ankle ROM, toes flexed

1. Flex or curl your toes all the way down. *(Image 12)*
2. Keep your toes curled, work your foot in full circles without letting your toes straighten out (this will be most difficult as you reach the bottom the circle). *(Images 13, 14)*

A set of 15 to 20 circles with your toes fully curled is the goal. Remember, if / when your foot cramps, extend the toes back to help release it!

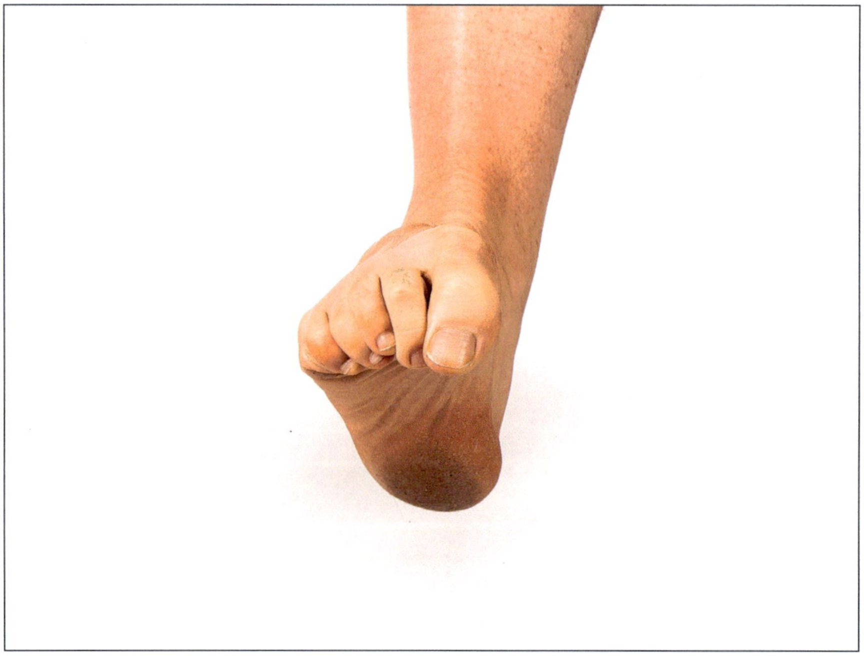

Image 12

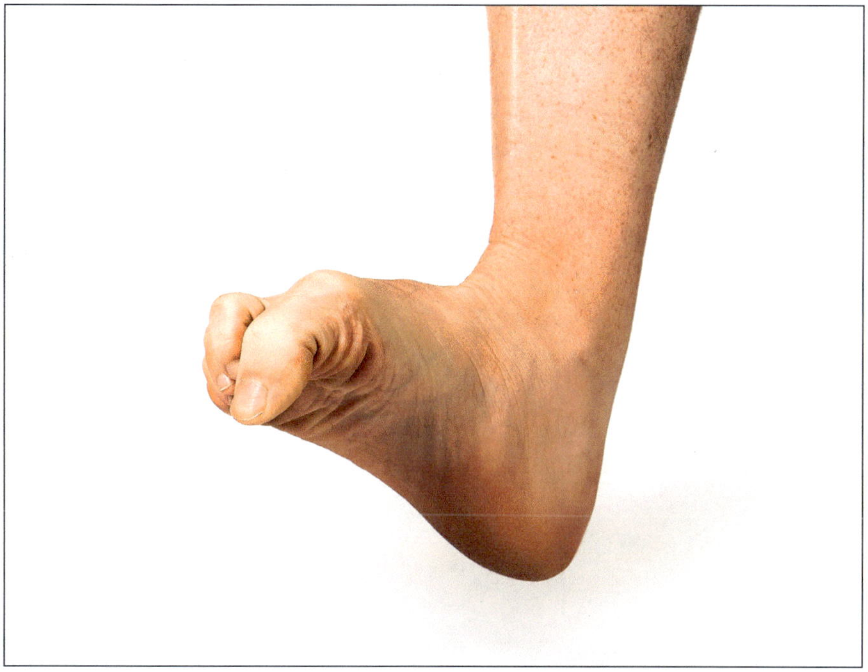

Image 13

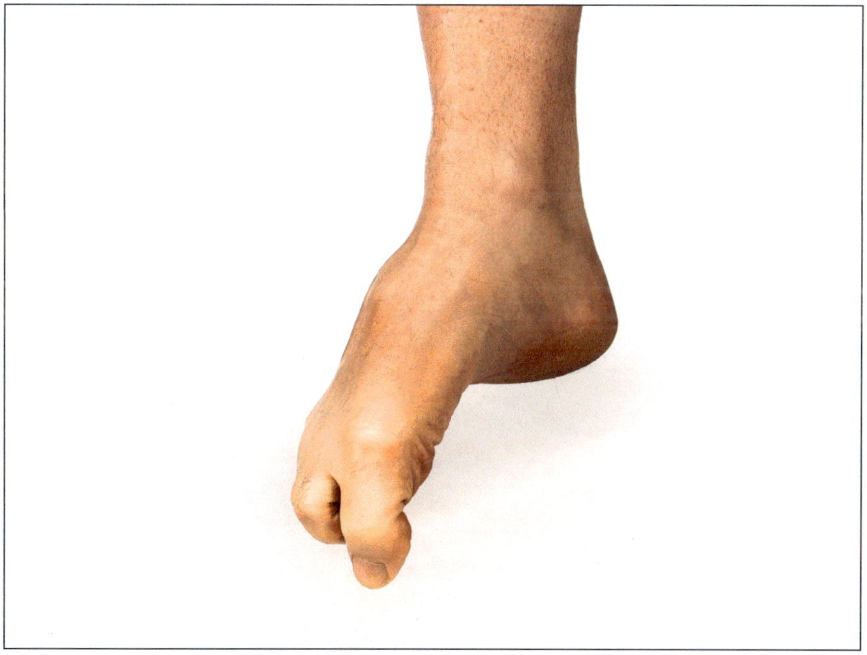

Image 14

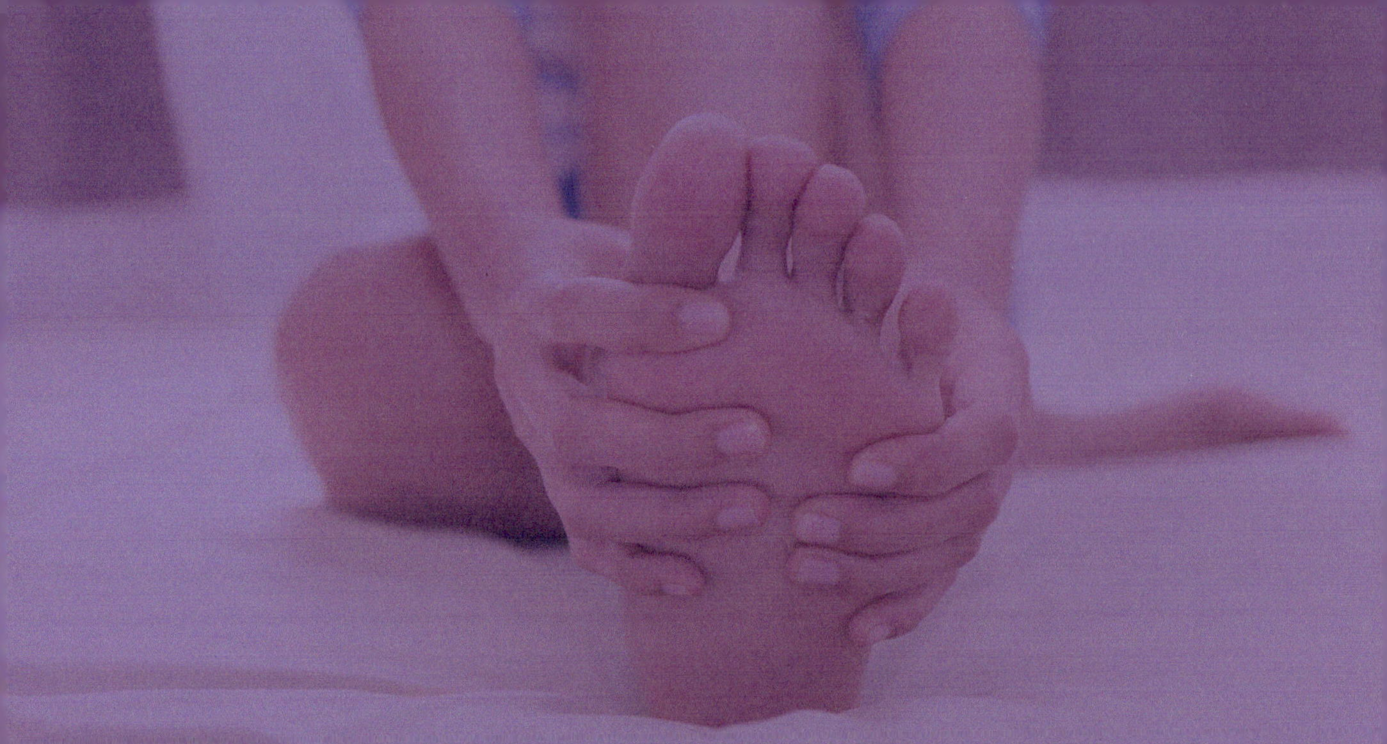
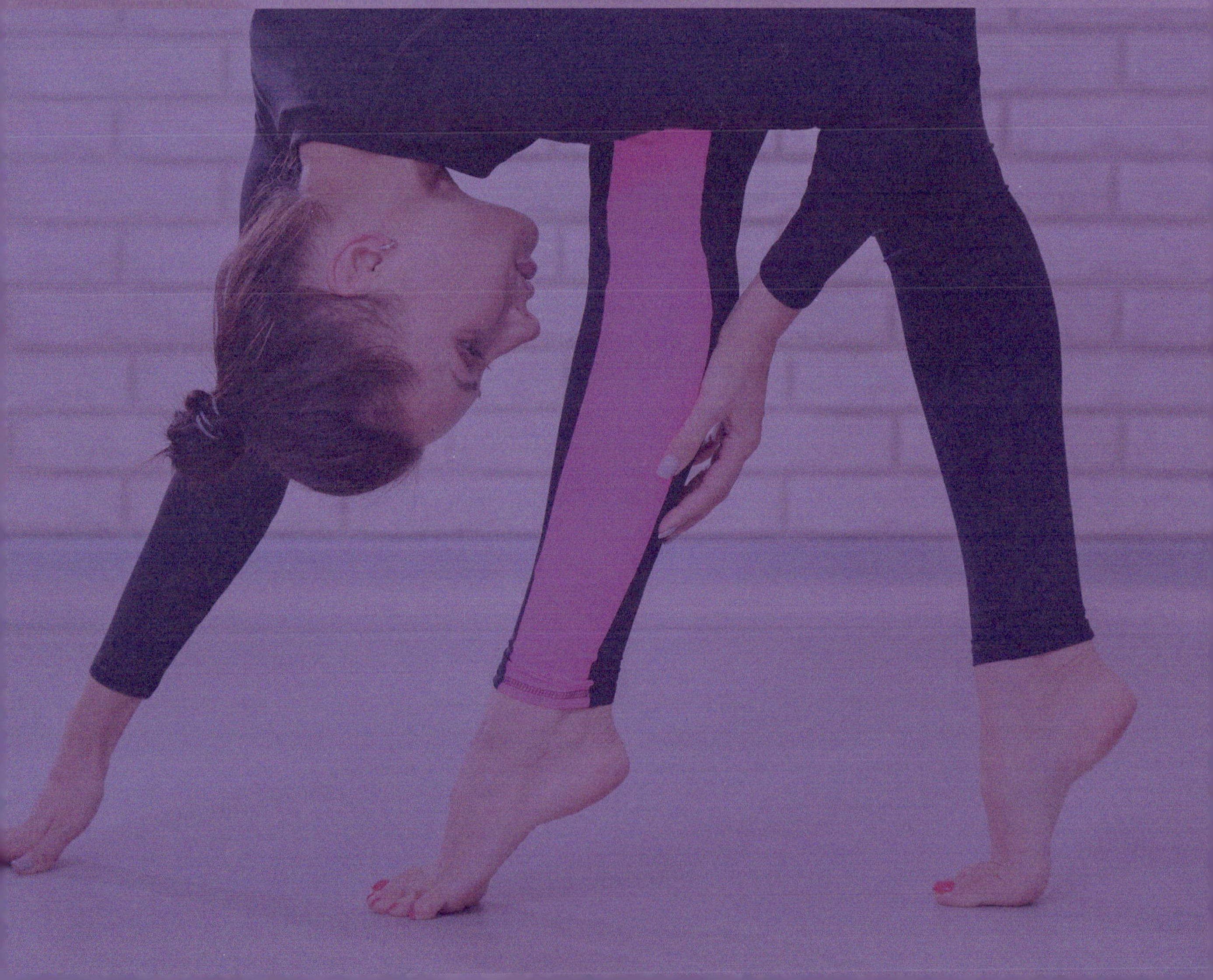

CHAPTER SIX

STEP TWO: INTRINSIC STRENGTHENING–THE SMALL STABILIZERS

Warm up–Alphabet

- Using your big toe for guidance, slowly and purposefully draw the alphabet with your feet. Once or twice through is all you need to warm up everything to be ready to go.

With the exercises below, start with one exercise, one set of 10 repetitions. Once you're able to complete three full sets without pain or your foot cramping, add the next exercise. If you attempt to do everything listed here the first time, you run the risk of getting some seriously painful foot cramps.

The Main Exercise– The Short Foot Exercise

This exercise is also called doming or Janda's short foot. It is the basis of many other exercises we will talk about. Dr. Davis has suggested that the foot works like the pelvis, in that large, extrinsic muscles are the prime movers, whereas the smaller, intrinsic muscles provide stabilization to the bone structure. Once these smaller (intrinsic) muscles are tired in your feet, they are no longer able to provide the foot with the support it needs to stay springy and elastic. This can lead to a decrease in foot stiffness, and a loss of arch height. When evaluating the effects of the short foot exercise over a four to eight week period, Mulligan and Cook concluded that participants' arches dropped less and became more stiff (stiffness in this case is a good thing), while balance and reach tests improved in almost every direction (Mulligan, 2013).

Using the short foot exercise as described by Janda in the book *Rehabilitation of the Spine* as the basis of developing deep foot strength is integral to super strong feet. The short foot exercise is not intuitive or easy to perform the first time you try! Researchers have suggested a three-step process to get the hang of this tricky feat of neuromuscular control:

1. Passive modeling of the exercise with someone familiar with the maneuver helps put your foot into the proper position so that you understand the motion. This could be any specialist, kinesiologist, etc. or simply a friend who has mastered the movement. You'll only be able to use partial weight-bearing while someone is helping you.
2. Active-assisted modeling, in which the therapist still helps you through the range, but it involves your contracting

the muscles to help pull the foot into the proper short-foot position.

3. Once you and the specialist are confident that you have got the hang of it, you're free to do the exercise on your own.

The same group of researchers caution that mastery of this exercise can be difficult, even with specialist help. So don't give up!

To that end, active-assisted modeling can be effective when neuromuscular stimulation is added. Electro-stimulation pads are placed on the foot, and when a small current is applied, muscles contract. This has been proven effective in a three-week program, with three sessions per week. As little as a single 20-minute session has been shown to affect the main muscle we're targeting, the abductor hallucis, in a positive way. Physiotherapists are the most common specialists to offer this kind of therapy, but still others such as pedorthists and podiatrists may offer it as well. If you're struggling with the short foot exercise, or if your foot muscles are very weak, this might be a good option for you.

EXERCISE:

The Short Foot Exercise

There will be a progression in this exercise, but to begin, try this:

1. Sit in a chair with your foot flat on the floor.
2. Point your feet straight ahead, ensuring that your foot is in a neutral position, neither pronated or supinated. *(Image 15)*

3. To rev up your arches, try to raise the arch of your foot by "scraping" the toes backward and contracting the muscles in the mid-back of the arch.

4. At the same time, keep the ball of your foot touching the floor. This may take some practice! *(Image 16)*

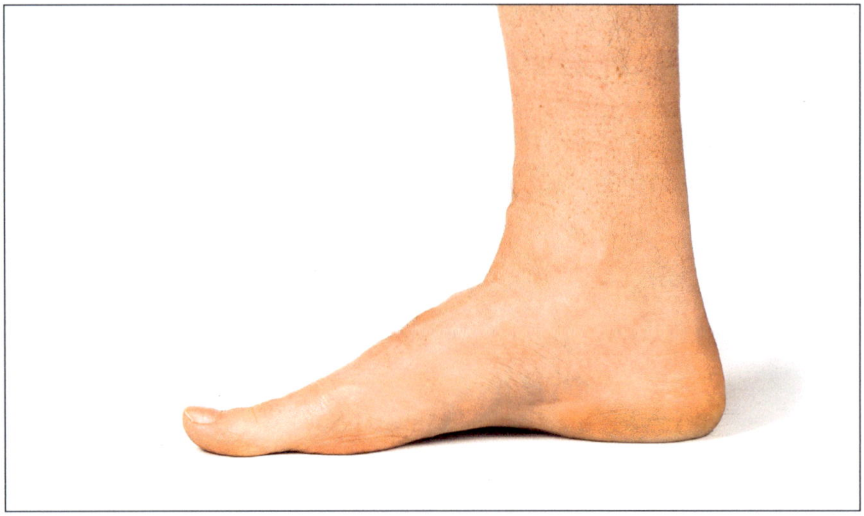

Image 15

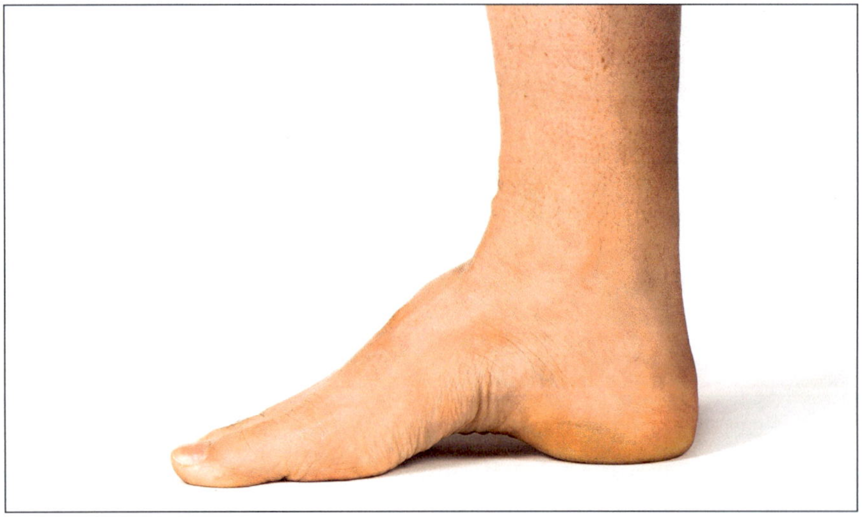

Image 16

Visit stuffaboutfeet.com to see the short foot exercise in action.

Repeat 10 times for each foot. If you're able to short foot out of the gate, great job! If not, it might take a few sessions. You could also contact a specialist for help modeling the exercise.

Need a little more help? There is some evidence, albeit mild, to suggest that performing this exercise with an incline of 30 degrees (30 degrees passive ankle dorsiflexion) may help increase activation of the AH by as much as 10% (Heo et al, 2014).

From now on, throughout the book, I'll describe performing the best short foot that you can as "***rev (or reving) up your arches***"

Once that becomes easy, try these progressions:

STANDING DOMING

Stand up straight, feet facing forward and neutral, and rev up those arches. Hold tight for 6-10 seconds, and release. Repeat 10 times.

SINGLE LEG

Repeat all of the above standing on one leg.

ADVANCED MOVE—SHORT FOOT FALLING FORWARD

Stand up straight, feet facing forward. Rev up your arches. Keeping your legs straight, slowly lean forward as far as you can go. Use your short foot, contracted hard, to brace your body and to pull it back up. *(Images 17, 18)*

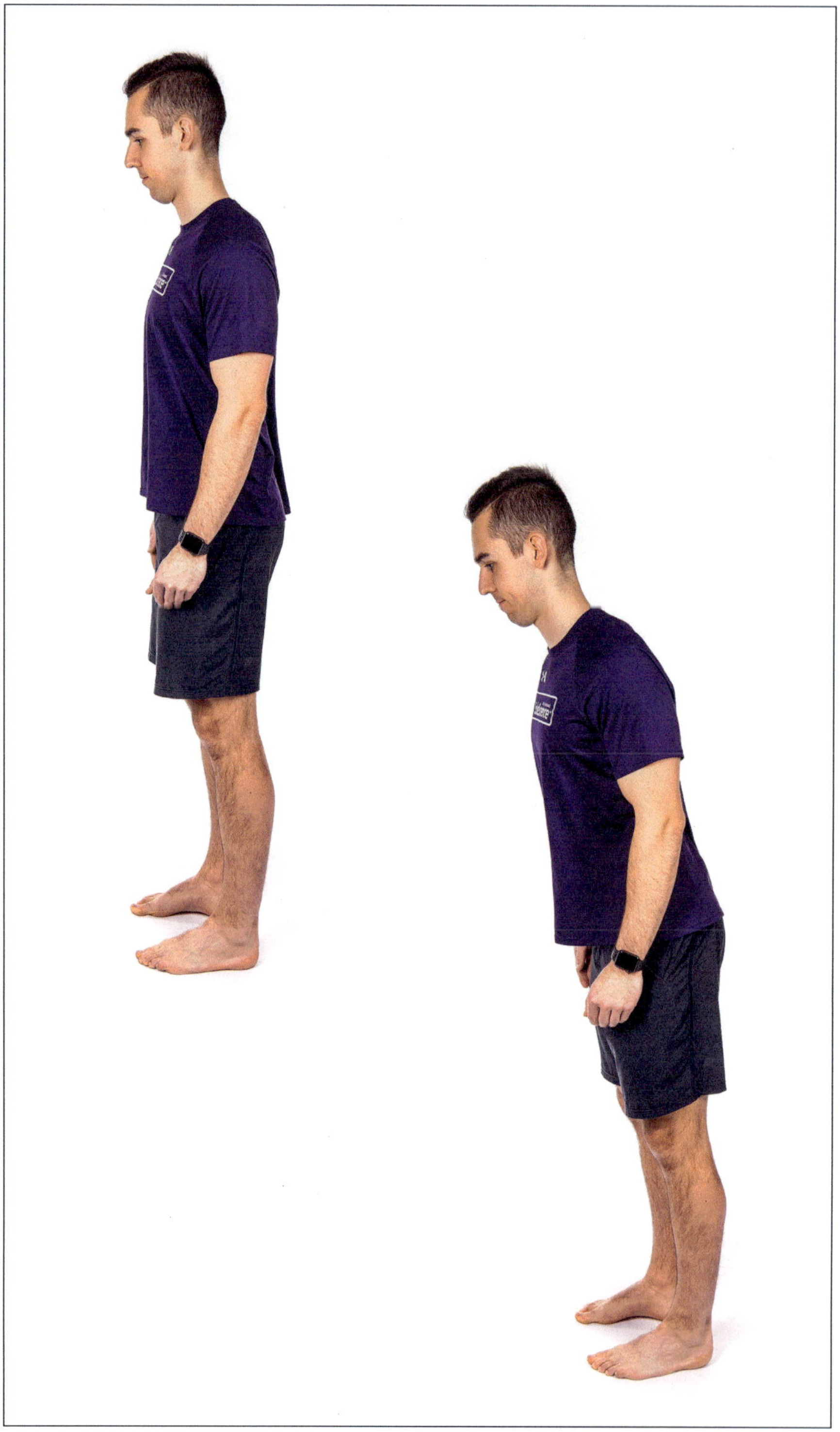

Images 17, 18

Foot-type-specific Recommendations for the Short Foot

EXTREMELY FLAT FEET

If your feet are of the pancake flat variety, as in when you walk barefoot on a wet surface there is almost a suction cup sound as your foot leaves the floor, this might apply to you. Often, this type of foot is unstable, lacking in range of motion, or with too much range. The main muscle we're targeting with the short foot is the abductor hallucis, and its main function is to support the arch on the inside (medial) side of your foot—that's a tall order when you don't have an arch.

I've had success with either a light, stretchy tape, like K-tape, in the arch to "lift" it or by externally rotating the lower extremity to lift the inside arch up. To see this in action, go to the video section of stuffaboutfeet.com/videos.

Try both and find which one works best. It has been suggested that custom foot orthoses for flat feet can work to strengthen the AH. By incorporating the short foot exercise and custom foot orthoses, individuals with extremely flat feet may be able to get stronger on this stabilizer muscle than without the orthoses (Jung, 2011).

DO BUNIONS AFFECT THE SHORT FOOT?

Bunions are the irregular position of two regular-shaped bones that produce a bump on the side of your toe. Can they affect your ability to perform some of these exercises? Yup, sure do. When the big toe has deviated, the AH is altered in its ability to pull in the proper direction. This gets worse as the deformity worsens. One researcher, Dr. Ward Glasoe, has proposed that strengthening of the AH may be a treatment in the conservative management of hallux valgus, and although no studies have proven that, yet, it certainly can't hurt to start, seeing that surgery is often the final treatment.

To properly activate the AH during the short foot, try using a small piece of tape to better align the big toe. Spacers and special alignment socks like the Bunion Bootie or Sockwell bunion sock work well, too.

Get the Toes Moving Again

All too often in clinical practice, we see people who have lost the ability to move their toes. This can happen for a variety of reasons, but we need to work on getting the toes to move again. There are a few contraptions and devices for this, but I recommend just using your fingers and some pressure to move them apart. Beware of contraptions that are the same thickness around all your toes. The spaces between your smaller toes are narrower than those between your large toes. I've seen patients who have torn their stabilizing intermetatarsal ligaments / joint capsule from exerting too much pressure with contraptions not designed with human ergonomics in mind, or by spreading their toes with too much force, too quickly. If you already have good range of motion and can move your toes well, toe sepertors, or even your fingers inbetween your toes can work just fine.

To get the toes moving try this:

EXERCISE:

Toe spreads

1. Use your fingers or a gel toe seperator, or even pedicure spacers, to seperate your toes depending on your comfort. *(Image 19)*

2. Twist your foot from side to side. This is a great stretch for the dorsal (top of the foot) fascia and will help get the toes moving again.

3. Curl your toes downward, extend them back, and spread them apart.

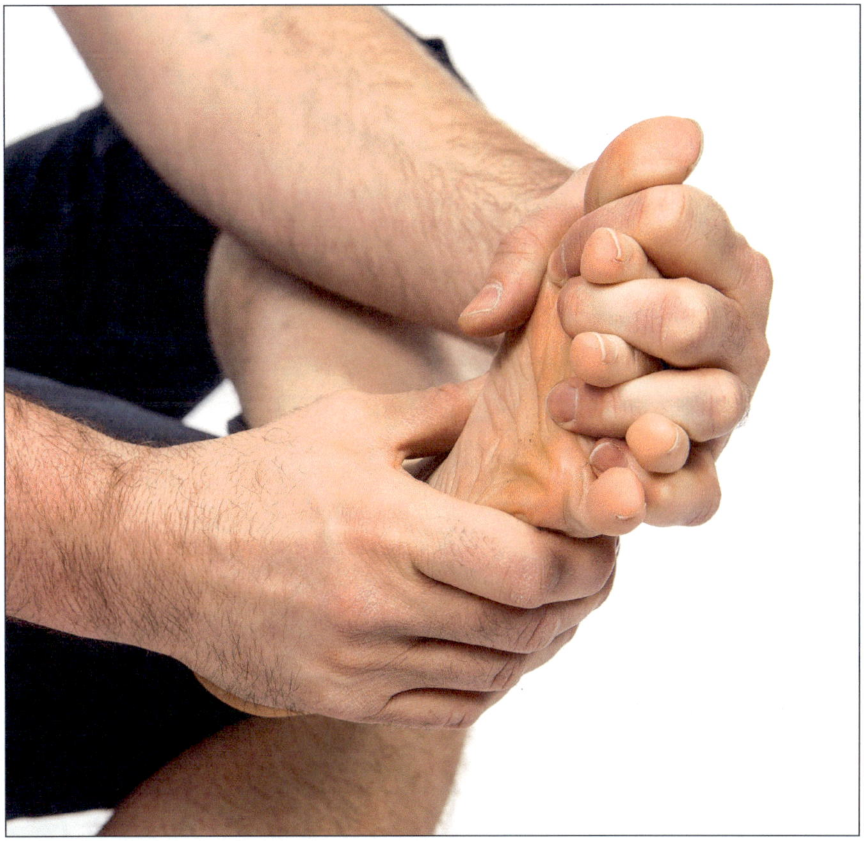

Image 19

While spreading them, try and contract the muscles deep in-between your toes (lumbricals) to start training them. This is a way to move your toes again. As you move them more and contract the muscles, you train your brain to send messages to the muscles to turn them on, and it will become easier to just contract without using your fingers. This will take some time and practice if your toes are stuck together, so hang in there! A word of caution (just like above)—don't force the toes apart. Ease into the spreading so that you don't get a small tear. Once you're able to spread your toes apart, the exercise below will become easier.

4. With your foot flat, try to spread your smaller toes as evenly as you can. *(Images 20, 21)*

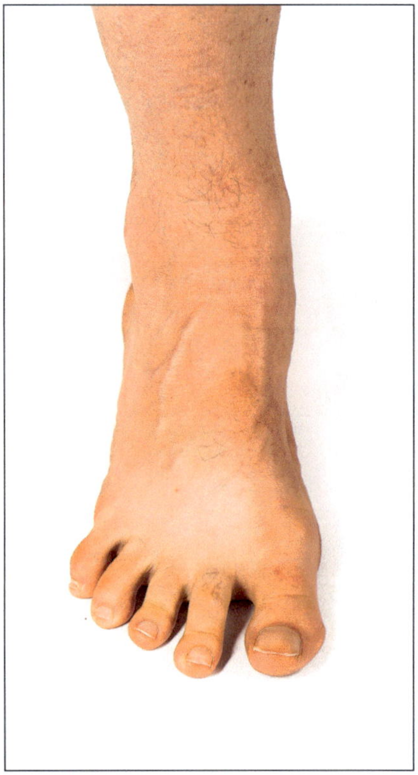

Image 20

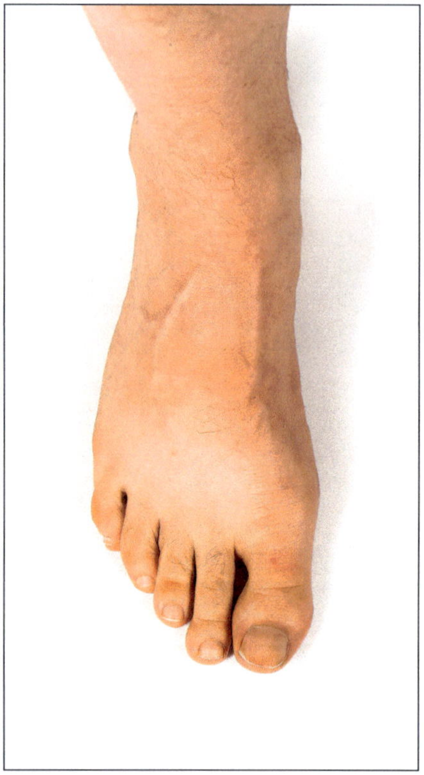

Image 21

EXERCISE:

Toe adduction

Adduction means pulling the toes together toward the center-line of your foot.

1. Sit in a chair and place pedicure separators between your smaller toes. (You can get these at any pharmacy.)
2. Pull your toes together. Hold for two seconds, then push your toes apart, hold for two seconds, and then relax for five seconds. To avoid cramping, start with just a few repetitions for each foot. Over a couple of weeks, work your way up to 10 repetitions for each foot. *(Images 22, 23)*

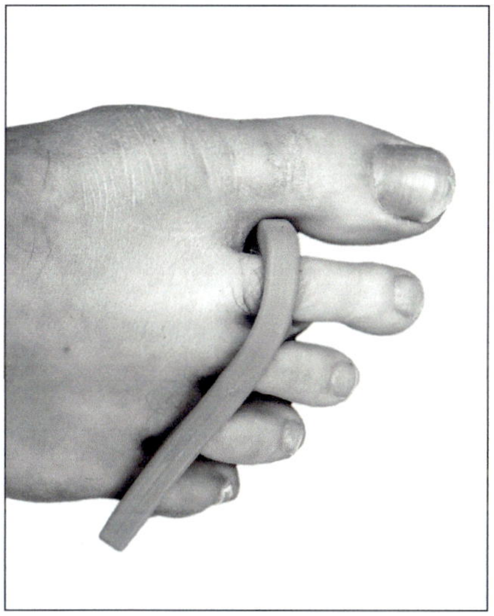

Image 22

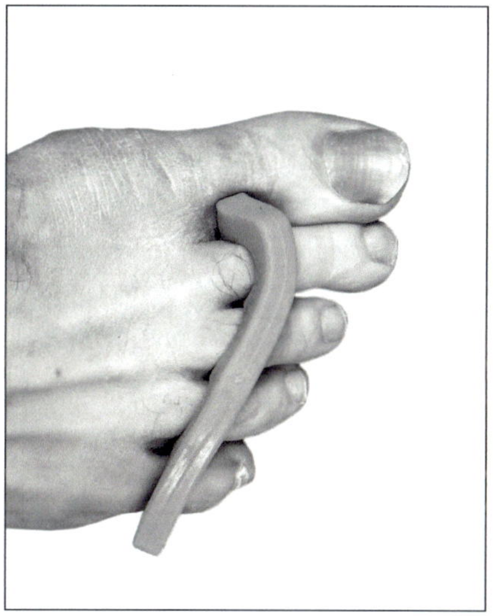

Image 23

ADVANCED MOVE

Are you ready to play some Rachmaninoff with your feet? Awesome. Try this one if the above is too easy:

EXERCISE:

Fifth toe adduction only

1. Lightly press your smaller toes into the ground, then activate, and move just your fifth toe away from your fourth toe.
2. Hold for 2–4 seconds, and bring it back. This is a neuromuscular control exercise and is maddeningly hard to get a hang of. If you simply can't spread your toes, go back to page 54 to read about getting your toes moving again and start there. *(Images 24, 25)*

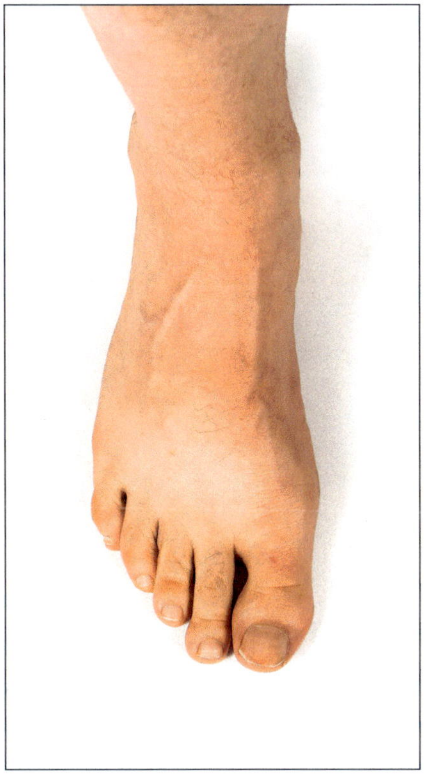

Image 24

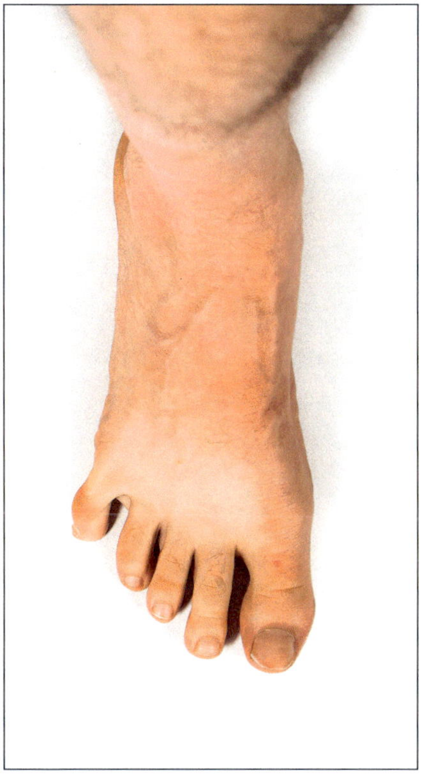

Image 25

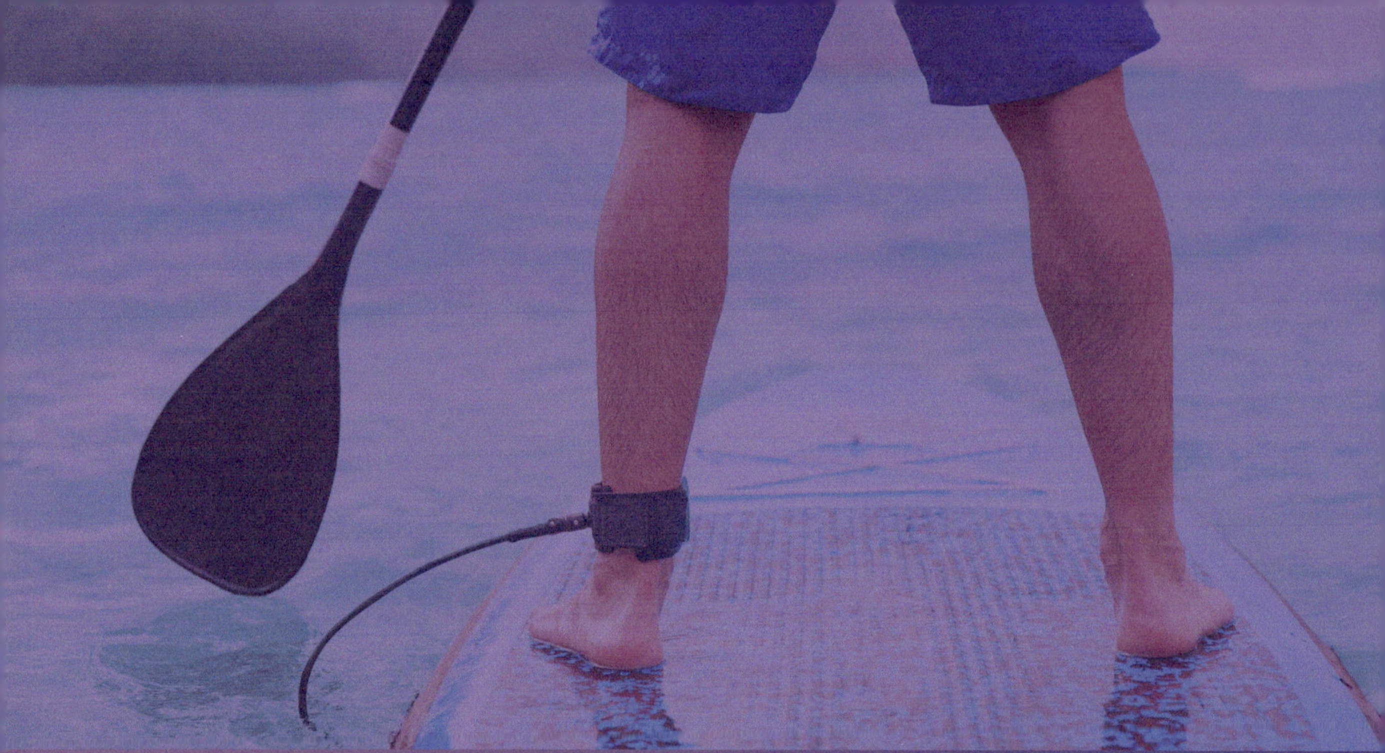
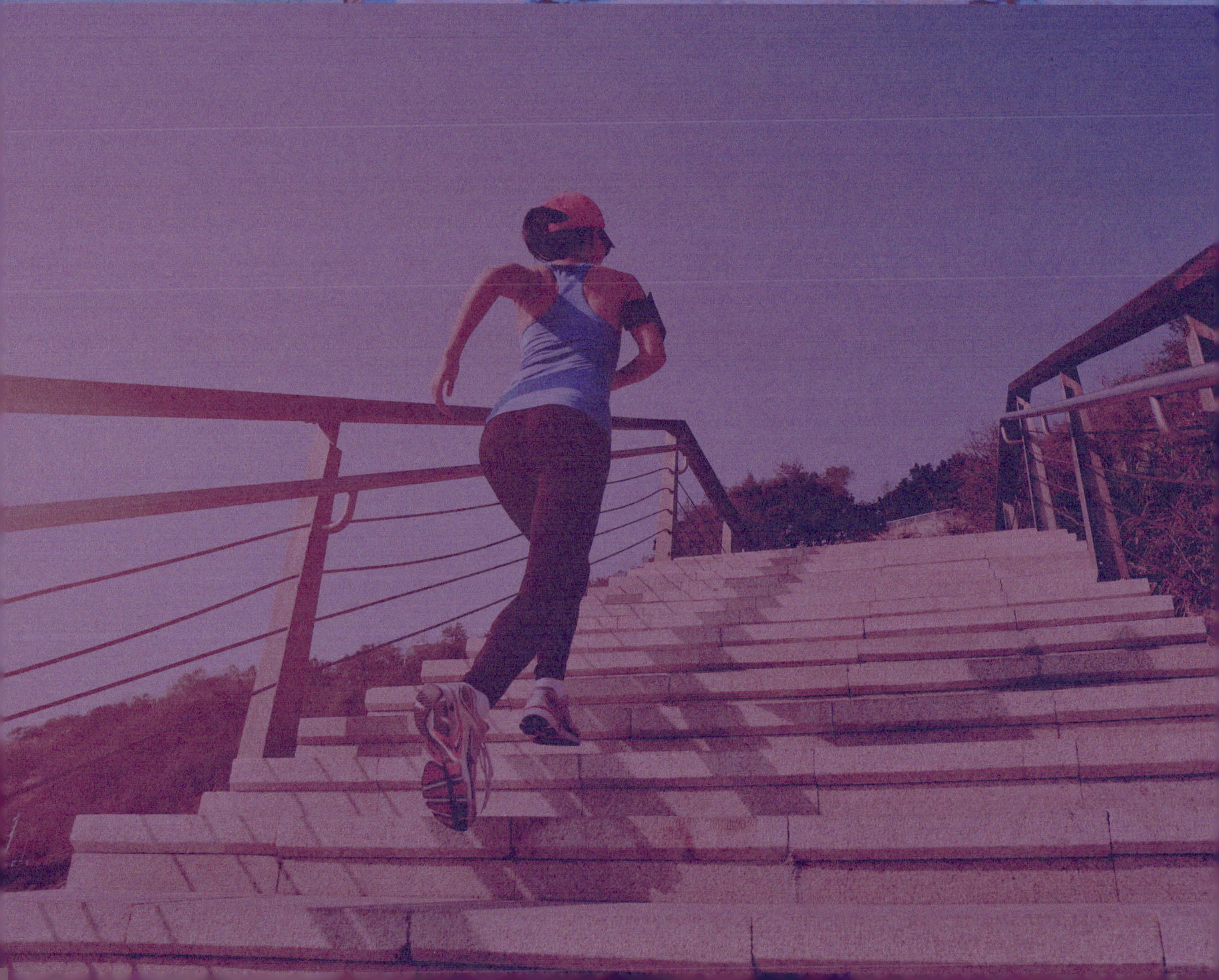

CHAPTER SEVEN

STEP THREE: EXTRINSIC MUSCLES–MAIN MOVER

EXERCISE:

Toe keyboard

In this external mover control exercise, the focus is to play an imaginary keyboard with either your big toe or your smaller toes. If you're having trouble getting the movement down, you can use your hands to assist getting started.

1. Lightly press the smaller toes into the ground and lift the big toe. *(Image 26)*

(continued)

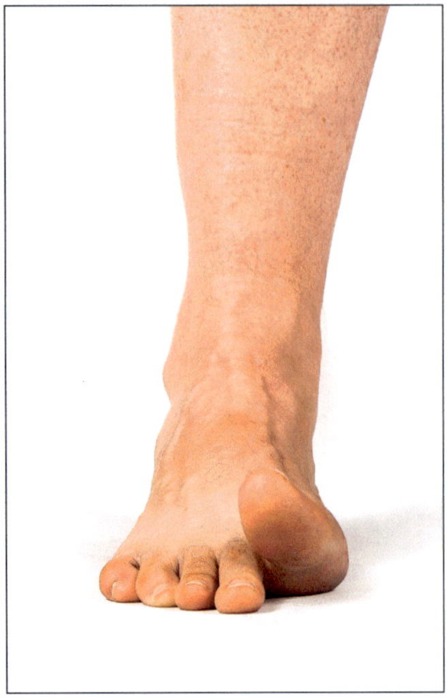

Image 26

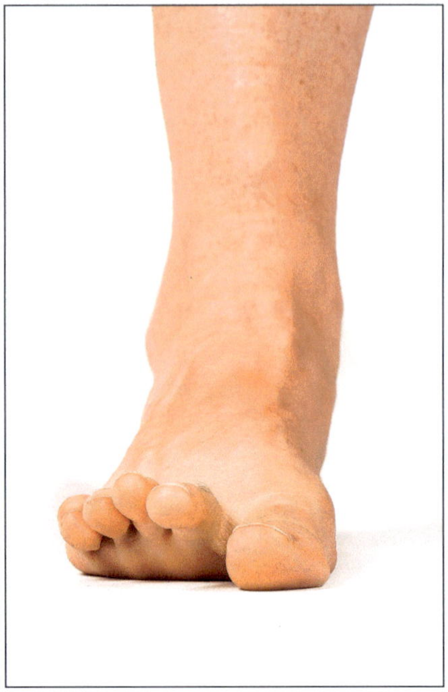

Image 27

2. Lightly press the big toe into the ground and lift the smaller toes. *(Image 27)*
3. Alternate back and forth between the two, 10 times each.

EXERCISE:

Towel crunch

You need a small towel for this exercise. *(Image 28)*

1. Place the towel on the floor.
2. Sit in a chair and place your foot on the towel.
3. Flex your toes hard enough to bunch up the towel.
4. Hold for two seconds and then relax for five seconds. Repeat 10 times for each foot.

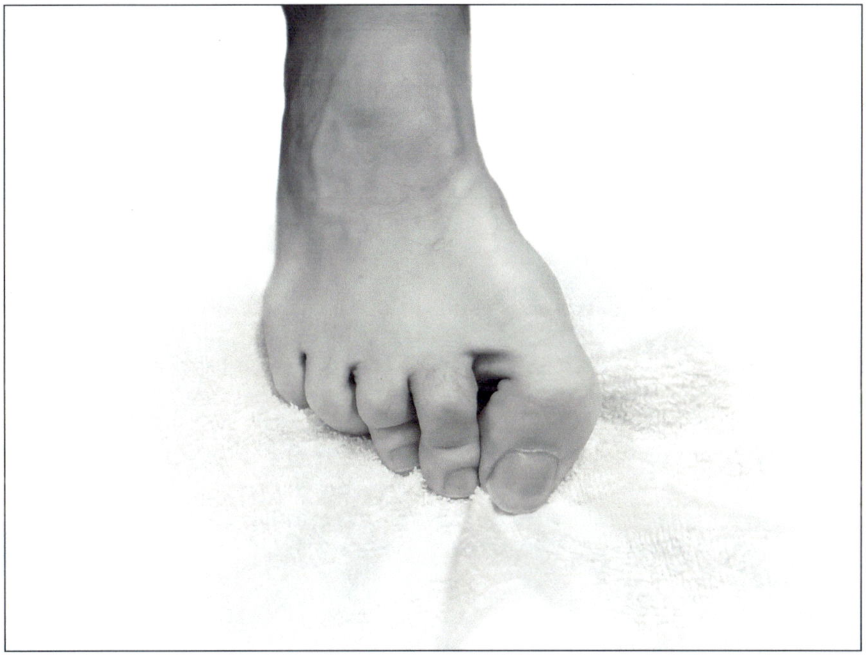

Image 28

ANKLE STABILITY

The exercises suggested here will work to increase strength in the muscles that support the ankle.

EXERCISE:

Band strengthening

1. Place a stretchy band around the inside of the foot.
2. Move the sole of your foot toward the inside, moving only at the ankle. *(Image 29)*
3. Pull inward, rotating from the ankle to strengthen the tib post (inside lower leg)
4. Reverse to strengthen peroneals (outer lower leg). *(Image 30)*

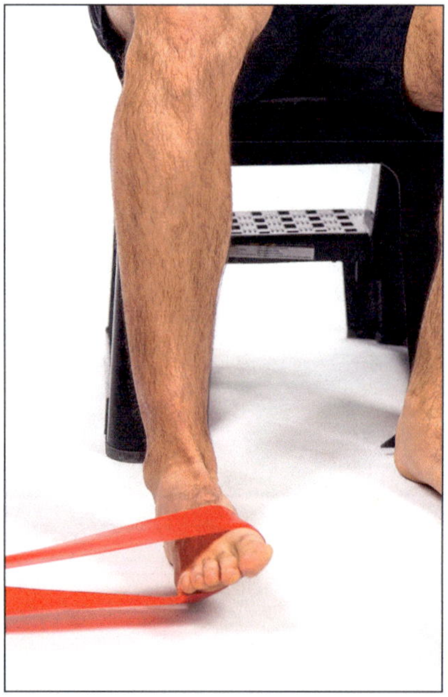

Image 29

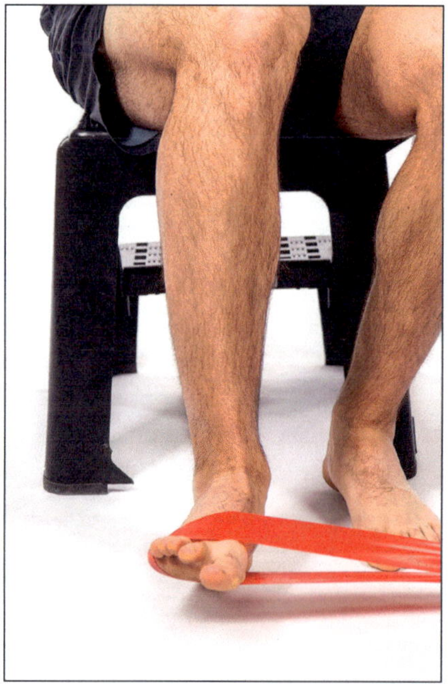

Image 30

EXERCISE:

Plantar flexors

1. Roll a small towel and place under the toes on a step. Hold onto a railing for support, but not so much as to make the exercise easier.
2. With both feet, raise up as far as you can go in a slow, controlled movement, three seconds up, three seconds down with a two-second pause at the top.
3. Once at the top of the movement, lift one leg, and with the other lower the heel down as far as it can go.
4. Start with no weight, and aim for one set of 12 reps.
5. Repeat on the other leg.
6. Once one set is easy, progress to 2, then 3.
7. Once three sets are easy, add weight by wearing a backpack filled with small hand weights, or books to make this exercise more challenging.

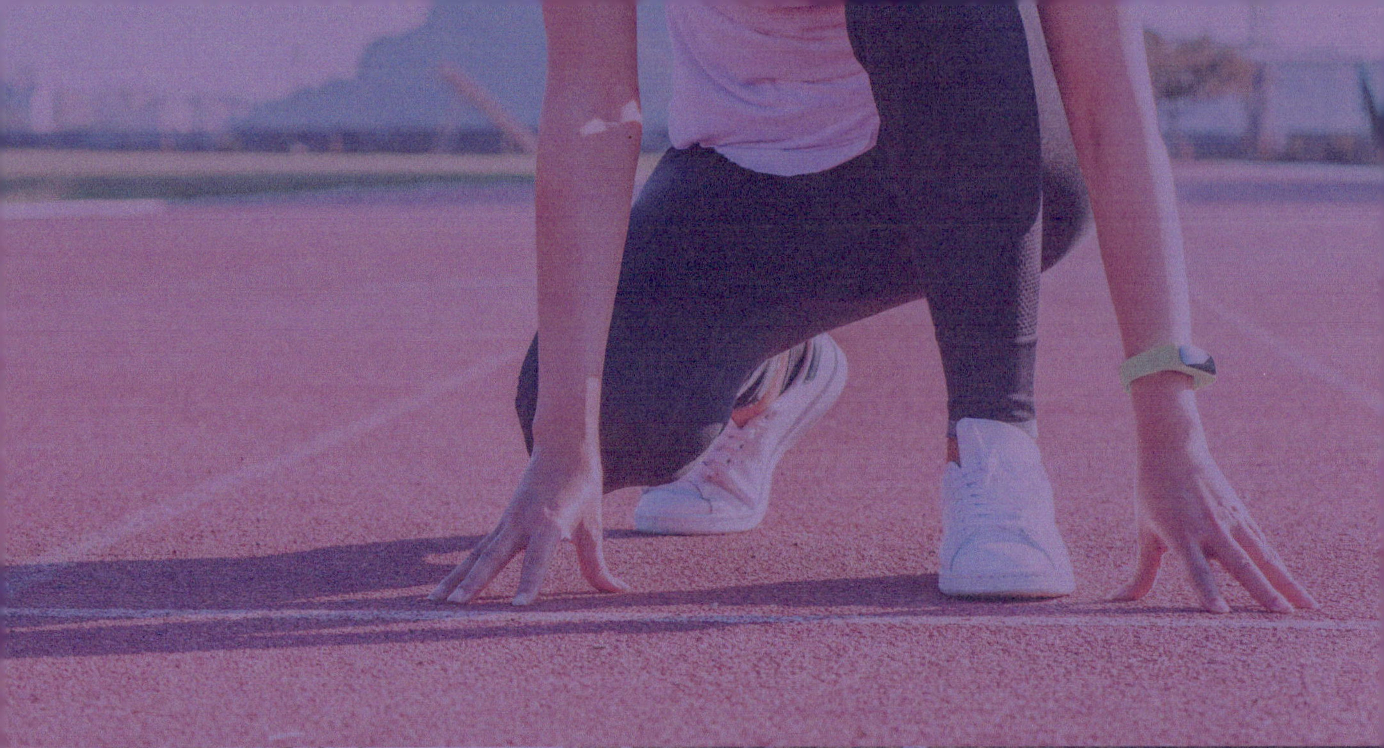

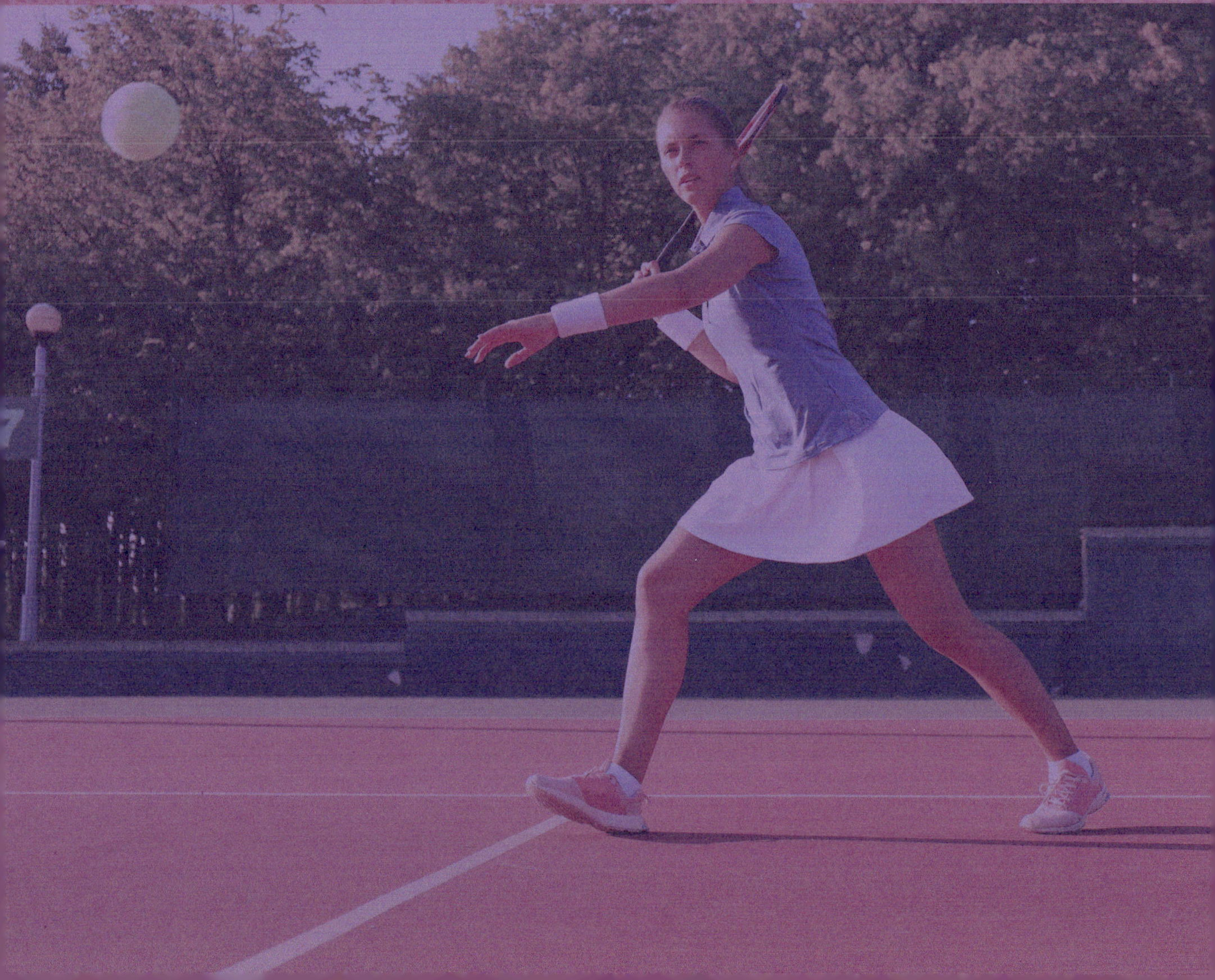

CHAPTER EIGHT

STEP FOUR: INCREASE YOUR BALANCE

Below is a simple balance protocol. If the suggested exercises are too easy and you're in need of something more substantial, I'd suggest talking with your physiotherapist. In 2012, Kelly et al showed that the intrinsic foot muscles are recruited when the demands of medial / lateral sway increased during single leg stance (standing on one leg). The research showed that while the smaller muscles in your feet are active during quiet standing, they increased their activation as demands to posture increased.

1. Stand on one foot, eyes open, looking straight ahead. Rev up your arch for foot stability. *(Image 31)*
2. Try to maintain balance (don't let your foot flop from side to side). Hold on to something to regain balance if needed, such as a doorway.

3. Hold for one to two minutes.

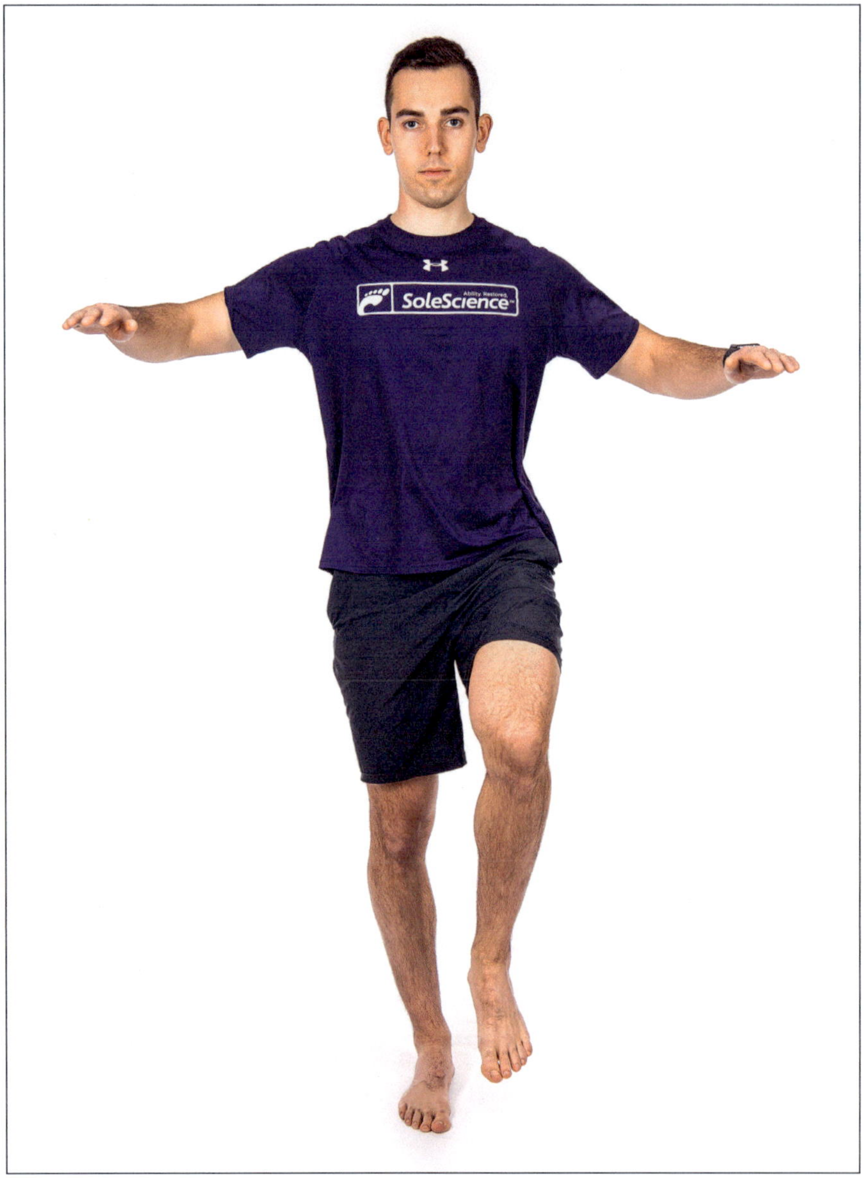

Image 31

4. Once this becomes easy, cross arms. Hold for one to two minutes. *(Image 32)*

5. Once this becomes easy too, close your eyes, and hold for one to two minutes. *(Image 33)*

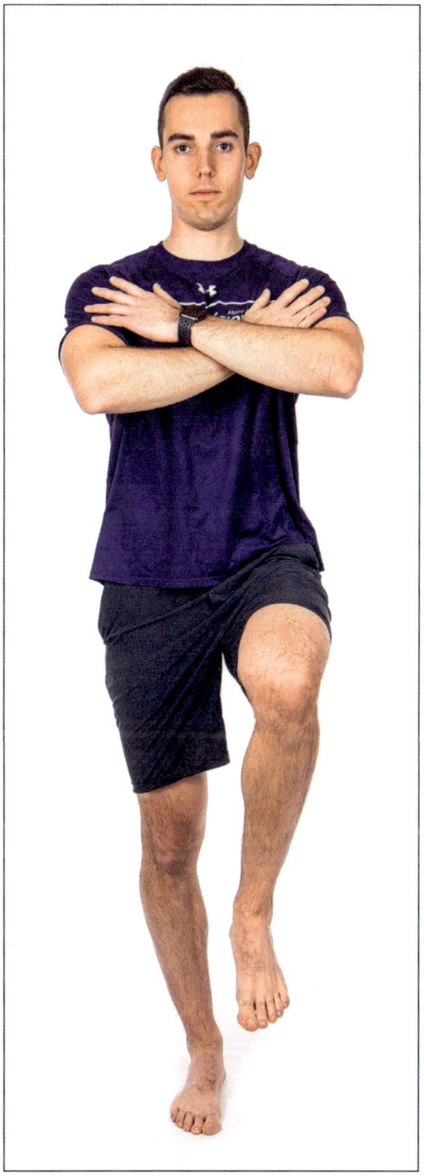

Image 32

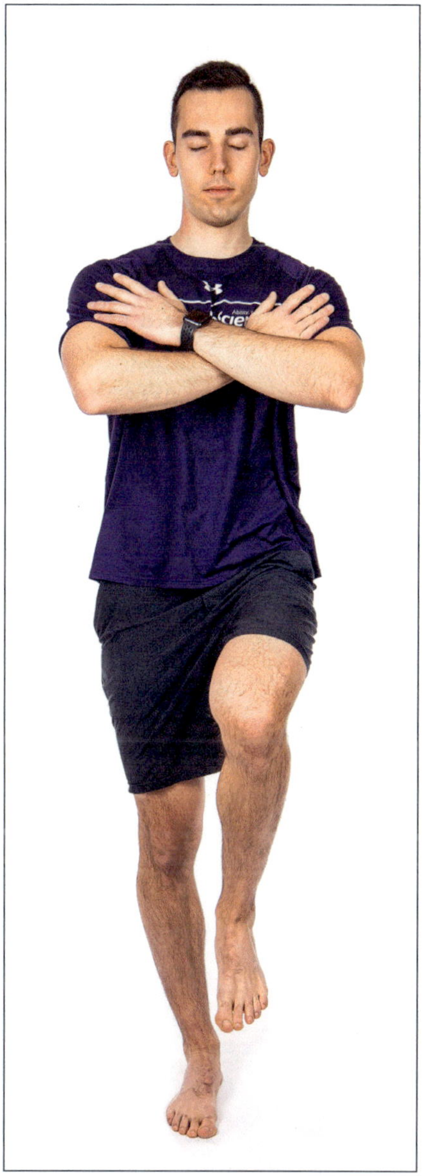

Image 33

6. Once all of it becomes easy, try de-stabilizing to stabilize. Do the exercise on a shallow pillow as a progression. *(Image 34)* *Note that it may take up to four to six weeks to progress all the way.

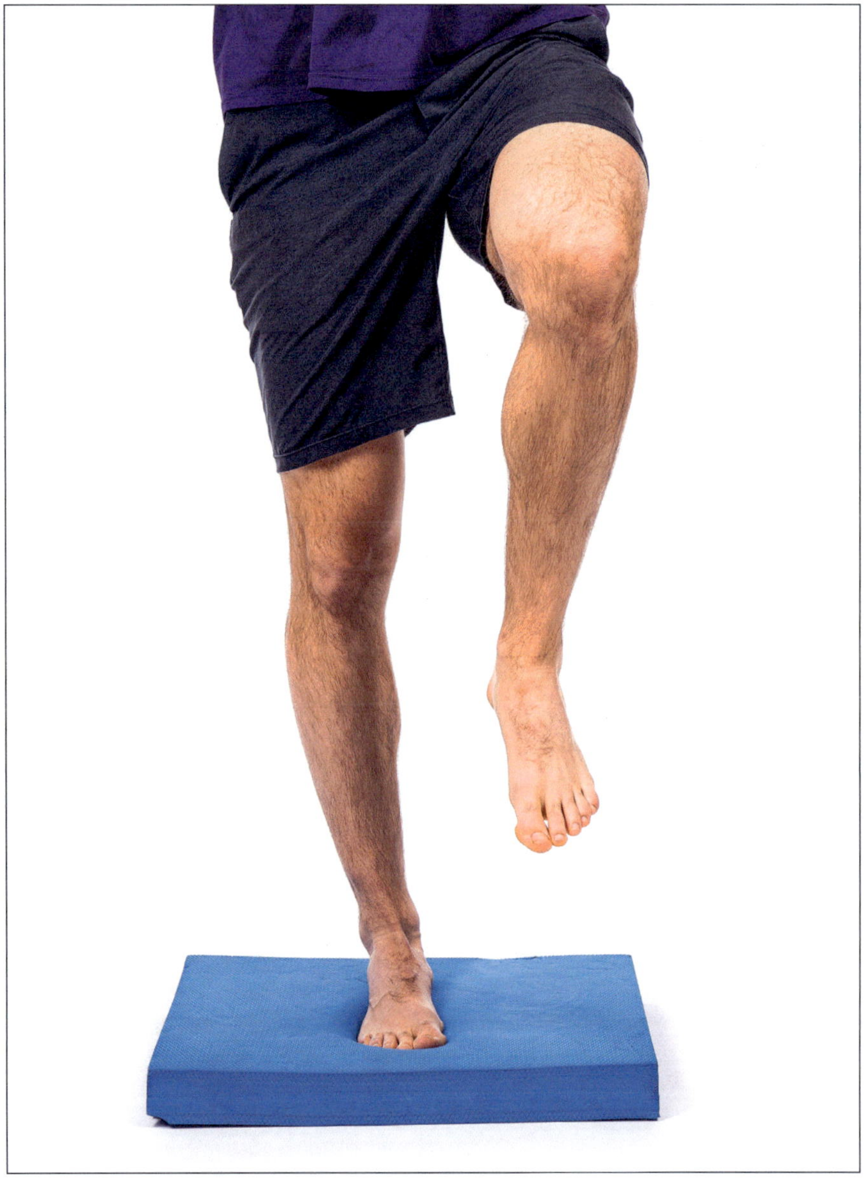

Image 34

ADVANCED BALANCE—SINGLE LEG, FOOT ROLL UP

Stand on one leg, rev up your arch with a short foot, hold your balance for five seconds, then roll up onto your forefoot while maintaining a stable foot. Lower. Repeat 10 times.

ADVANCED—SINGLE LEG HOPS AND SHORT FOOT

How do you know when you're close to seriously strong feet? Can you do everything in the previous pages and think to yourself, "C'mon man, what else can you throw at me?" Try this. Special thanks to Dr. Davis for this one!

Stand on one leg, rev up your arches, balance for five seconds, then hop. How many times can you do it? 10, 25, ... 75 before you fall to the floor in a whimpering mess, doubled over clutching your calves that have all cramped up?

Want to make that even more difficult? Do it while skipping, or throwing a ball, or some version of an exercise where you need to perform a repetitive task with your arches are reved up.

Seriously, that's a good test of solid, healthy feet.

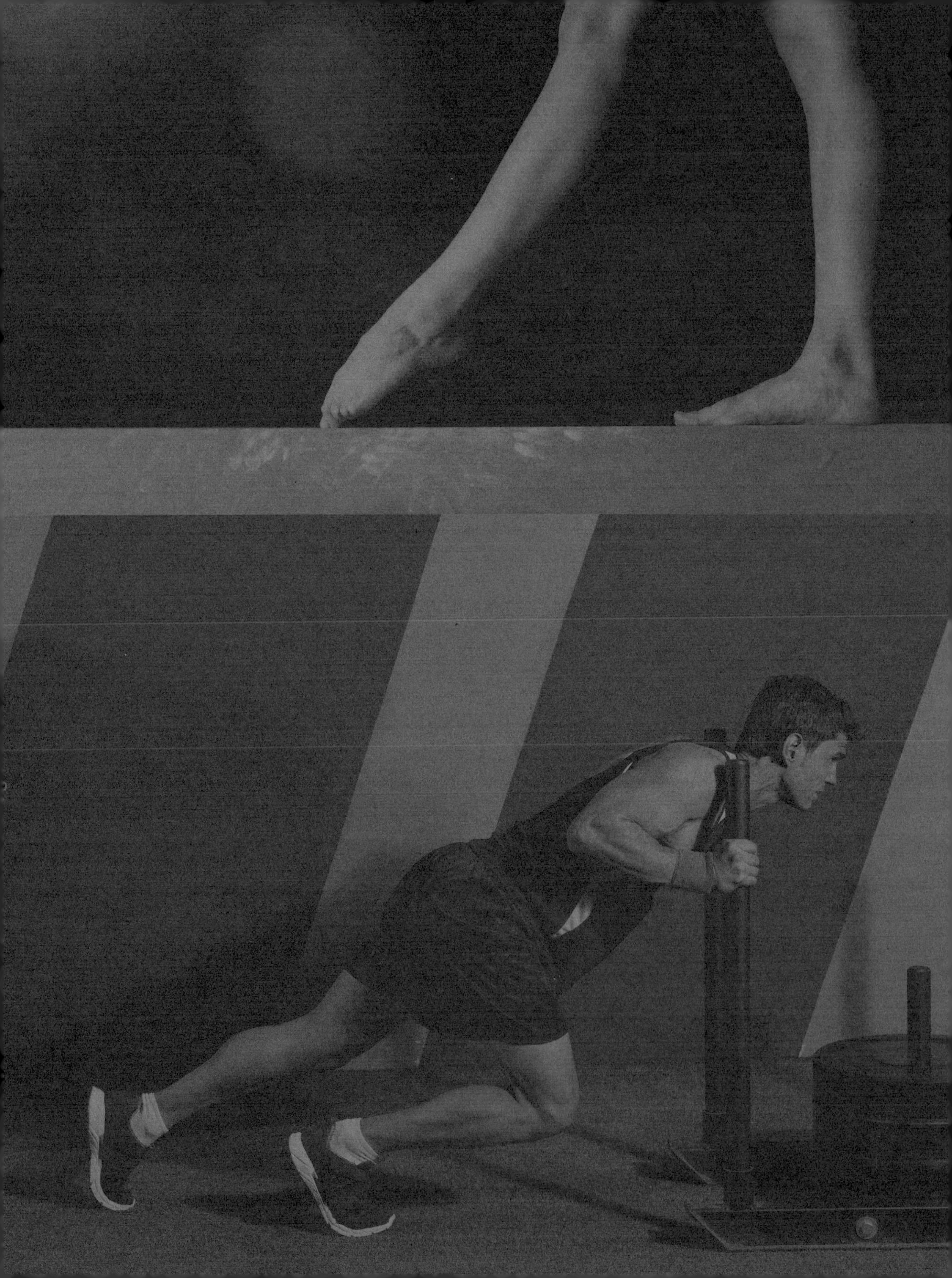

CHAPTER NINE

STEP FIVE: DYNAMIC STABILITY

Once you have the strength exercise mastered in Step Four, the dynamic ones presented here will help keep your foot and ankle stable while you perform more dynamic movements. A stronger base of support can only serve to help performance.

EXERCISE:

Single leg, short foot ball throw

1. Stand on one leg, rev up your arch, and hold your balance for five seconds.
2. Then throw a ball at a hard surface or rebounder. Hold yourself steady while maintaining a stable foot to catch it. Repeat 10 times.

EXERCISE:

Single leg ball twists

1. Stand up straight, feet facing forward and neutral, rev up those arches.
2. Hold tight for three to six seconds, then twist your torso keeping your core tight, or pass the ball to someone behind you. Repeat 10 times.

EXERCISE:

Single leg touchdowns

1. Stand up straight, feet facing forward and neutral, and rev up those arches.
2. Hold tight for three to six seconds, keeping your core tight, then bend at the waist to touch the floor. Repeat 10 times

EXERCISE:

Ladder hops

1. With a flat, fabric, ladder on the floor in front of you, perform a single leg short foot.
2. Hop from rung to rung on the floor, keeping your foot as contracted as possible to help make your foot rigid at push off and act as a spring while you land and remember to keep your core tight.

3. Before the next hop, if you've lost a tight short foot, relax, re-contract and hop again.
4. Repeat with the other foot. Don't have a fancy ladder? Try placing flattened paper towel rolls spaced out like one.

EXERCISE:

Hop downs from step

1. Standing on a raised surface no higher than six to eight inches, perform a short foot.
2. Hop off the raised surface and land with the foot contracted. The goal here is to use the contracted short foot to absorb the shock of landing. Your foot will naturally lower to absorb the load.

EXERCISE:

Single leg squat

Can you hold your arches reved up while performing a single leg squat?

1. Stand on one leg. Rev up your arch and hold for three to six seconds.
2. Once your foot is not twitching trying to find its balance, bend your knee and perform a single leg squat, focusing on keeping the short foot.

EXERCISE:

Single leg heel raise

1. Stand on one leg. Rev up your arch and hold for three to six seconds.
2. Once your foot is not twitching trying to find its balance, roll up slowly into a full call raise, hold for one second at the top, and slowly lower back to the floor.

Working the Short Foot into Your Daily Life

Remember what Dr. Davis said in her interview?

> "You can incorporate doming into your everyday activities, such as while you're standing in line at the grocery store checkout. We teach people how to do active standing, which starts with the foot but also includes some gluteus maximus and lower abdominal activation. It's amazing how different their posture looks when people start to do this."

Enter Dr. Kelly Starrett. In his New York Times bestseller, *Becoming a Supple Leopard*, Dr. Starrett recommends the exact same "active standing" by reminding his athletes to "get organized" by keeping their feet pointed straight, Squeeze the butt muscles to bring the pelvis into alignment, turn their abs on to 20%, balancing the ribcage over the pelvis and the head and shoulders in a neutral position. The benefit, Starrett suggests, is a neutral spinal position, and it's from this position that a human finds their power. This a gross over-simplification of Starrett's method, and you really should check out **https://thereadystate.com** to see it in action.

Now That You're Stronger, What Kind of Shoes Should You Wear?

Recall that in the beginning of this book, I called attention to human variability. With that in mind, some people are going to rock minimal shoes, while it'll destroy others (this is also what I see daily in clinical practice, too). *There is no perfect shoe.*

So what is the "right" shoe for you? When you stand in awe of the footwear wall of your local sporting goods store, how do you know which is the best at minimizing your chance of injury? The short answer? I can't offer you "the best shoe." The vast variations in our individual feet, combined with what each of us finds comfortable, mixed with our unique anthropomorphic characteristics and movement patterns, makes it almost impossible for me to predict what you'll like the best. What I can do, though, is educate you on what to watch out for when buying, trying on, and using them to best arm you for a trip to the shoe store.

Research published in the *Journal of the American College of Sports Medicine* suggests individual dynamic testing, based on a study looking at different styles of shoes and their ability to cushion basketball players during a 60cm drop jump. The researchers concluded that while they could not predict which shoe would be the best for each player, it did seem as though some styles are better than others. The authors suggest that while materials testing can provide valuable information regarding shock absorption, it lacks the *individual performance of the player* who wants to wear that shoe.

Comfort

In scientific terms, 'comfort' as it relates to footwear selection has been described as "an ever-changing individual perception influenced by mechanical, neurophysiological and psychological factors" (Kryger et al, 2017) Or simply: *comfort is only comfortable to you.* It's not surprising that when asked, comfort is of paramount concern to athletes, however injury prevention was on the lower end of the priority scale. Odd. Uncomfortable footwear is not only associated with increased risk of injury (Kinchington,2012,) but has also been suggested to affect performance by way of increased fatigue!

Why in the world, then, would you not want your shoes to be as comfortable as possible? Time and time again, though, there seems to be this notion that "Oh, they'll break in" or "it's okay to blister, my shoes are new."

To blisters and break-in, I say , "heck no!". Comfort is what you should shoot for right out of the gate. There shouldn't be a trade off to allow them to break in. There are all kinds of ways an *experienced* shoe fitter can make shoes more comfortable—stretching, punching out, lifting, padding, lace changing, just to name a few. This is why I ALWAYS advocate for experienced shoe *fitters*, and not just undertrained shoe *fetchers* (those who just go to the back and say, "here you go.").

Minimal / Barefoot Shoes

Minimal and barefoot shoes are terms often used interchangeably, however they are two different styles of footwear. Both styles are meant to offer less than traditional support to mimic something close to being barefoot. A minimal shoe usually has a thin to moderate midsole, a low 0-6mm of heel height, and generally little to no support features. They're very, very flexible, so if you're a pronator, the shoe will allow you to continue to pronate. If you're a real supinator, it's going to allow you to continue to supinate. Barefoot shoes are those that offer little more than a foot covering between you and the ground. The shoe is really just meant to be a layer between your foot and the ground to provide some protection from the elements and the running surface.

As the benefits of barefoot running have become more controversial, these shoes have become less popular. Some people still say to me, "But dude, I *love* my barefoot shoes." And, "Didn't you see that Adebe Bikila won the Gold *barefoot*?" (in 1960, in Rome, where he posted a then world record of 2:15:16.) That's OK—keep wearing them. By now, I think you get the point that we're all different, and what works for one won't work for all. But some people try them and just hate them, or worse, get injured while wearing them. Oh, and as a side note the full story about Bikila is that he tried new shoes before the event that gave him blisters and so he chose to go barefoot. In fact, four years later, he ran for gold again in Tokyo and posted a ***better*** time [2:12:11.2], shod! But I digress...

I've seen some cases where people have improved with the use of barefoot shoes. The internet abounds with anecdotal cases of improvement. But I've also seen cases where people have received stress fractures from barefoot shoes. There's research to support both sides of the argument, and one side hasn't won out over the other—yet. If you don't have any injury problems and want to try barefoot shoes, go ahead. Personally and professionally, if you do have a history of injury, I don't advocate wearing minimal shoes without a long, slow breaking in period, and perhaps even a transition shoe, which has somewhere in between the traditional 8-12 mm heel and the 0-6mm of a minimal shoe. Research suggests that transition shoes ease the switch and may, in fact, lower the likelihood of new injury while trying to get used to a lower heel drop athletic shoe.

Why try minimalist shoes? There might be reasons these shoes can be beneficial for you, but you need to be aware of the pros and cons. Minimalist shoes were first designed to allow runners to experience running close to barefoot while still getting some basic protection from the elements and the environment. Wearing these shoes for drills, or while doing plyometrics or other short drills, may in fact help stretch muscles in both length and tension by putting your heels closer to the ground. The shoes may also force you to fatigue the smaller, deeper foot muscles, which will strengthen them. In fact, research done by Miller et al. suggests that this might be the case in minimal shoes. In a group of 33 healthy runners, these researchers studied the effects of training in a shoe with a heel of 4mm or less (New Balance Minimus 4mm, or the Merrell Pace Trail Glove 0mm) on the muscle cross sectional area and muscle volume of some of the muscles on the bottom of the foot and arch stiffness. They found that when compared to a 12mm, cushioned running shoe, the lower heel condition produced a significant difference in cross section and volume of two of the three muscles tested, suggesting that a 12-week program in lower heeled shoes resulted in stronger, more stiff arches.

Furthermore, Chen et al found that runners who were habitually shod, after transitioning to a barefoot (Vibram 5 fingers) shoe after a six-month training program to help them habituate to barefoot running, showed increases in both forefoot and rear-foot muscle group volume (measured by MRI) by 7-9%. (Chen et al. 2016)

Conversely, to the Miller findings, Ryan et al suggested that in runners preparing for a 10km event "running in minimalist footwear appears to increase the likelihood of experiencing an injury." (Ryan, 2013)

Malisoux et al concluded that the heel drop (or the offset between the heel and toes) did not affect injury risk in runners overall, while stratified analysis suggested that lower drop shoes may be more hazardous to regular runners, and preferable for occasional runners. (Malisoux, 2017) So you can see here that *even the best evidence is varied.*

The variability described earlier has its own risks, however. Some research suggests that lowering the heel with this type of footwear can increase the load on the Achilles tendon by as much as 38 %. This could lead to an injury. It may not be the best thing if you're experiencing a bout of Achilles tendinitis or have had other injuries in the past.

Remember the tissue stress curve from the first part of this book. Some people who fall on the right side of the curve will have no issue with going barefoot. They'll self-select to do well in this style of footwear. Others, who fall more on the left side of the curve, will try these shoes and get injured. I see this a lot in my sports medicine pedorthics practice. Even when these people make a real effort to ease into the minimalist protocol, they wind up with new aches and pains, or worse, a sidelining injury.

Interested in learning more? I wrote a book on athletic shoe selection called SoleSelection that you can find on Amazon.

Conclusion

By now, I'm sure that you understand two things:

1. To keep your feet healthy, you need to get and work at keeping them strong. You can use the short foot exercise throughout your day to challenge this.

2. There is not one simple solution for everyone. How you go about getting stronger and how you choose to select and use footwear, orthoses, and the exercises in this book will all vary, and that's perfectly okay.

If you've made it through the exercises here, you're probably feeling awesome and have a new-found sense of balance and strength. Do you find that other exercises are easier since you've strengthened your feet? Drop me a line at colin@stuffaboutfeet.com and let me know! Or if you have your own exercise you'd like me to consider for the second edition of this book, I'd love to see it.

To your health!

Colin

BIBLIOGRAPHY

Alexander, I. J. (1997). The Foot: Examination & Diagnosis (2nd ed.). Churchill Livingstone.

Balsdon, M. E. R., Bushey, K. M., Dombroski, C. E., Lebel, M.-E., & Jenkyn, T. R. (2016). Medial Longitudinal Arch Angle Presents Significant Differences Between Foot Types: A Biplane Fluoroscopy Study. *Journal of Biomechanical Engineering*, 138(10), 1-6.

Balsdon, M. E. R., Dombroski, C. E., Bushey, K. M., & Jenkyn, T. R. (2019). Hard, soft and off-the-shelf foot orthoses and their effect on the angle of the medial longitudinal arch: A biplane fluoroscopy study. *Prosthetics and Orthotics International,* 43(3), 331-338.

Balsdon, M. E. R., Dombroski, C. E., Bushey, K. M., & Jenkyn, T. R. (2021). Impression Methods for Custom Foot Orthoses – Comparing Semi-Weight-Bearing Foam and Non-Weight-Bearing Plaster using a Kinematic Measurement of the Medial Longitudinal Arch. *Journal of Prosthetics and Orthotics,* 33(1), 26-33.

Body Composition of Adults, 2012 to 2013. (2015). Retrieved from http://www.statcan.gc.ca/pub/82-625-x/2014001/article/14104-eng.htm

Bolívar, Y. A., Munuera, P. V, & Padillo, J. P. (2013). Relationship between tightness of the posterior muscles of the lower limb and plantar fasciitis. *Foot & Ankle International*, 34(1), 42–48.

Burns, J., Landorf, K. B., Ryan, M., Crosbie, J., & Ouvrier, R. (2007). Interventions for the prevention and treatment of pes cavus (high-arched foot deformity). *Cochrane Database Systematic Reviews*, (4), 8–10.

Chevalier, T. L., & Chockalingam, N. (2012). Effects of foot orthoses: How important is the practitioner? *Gait and Posture*, 35(3), 383–388.

Chundru, U., Liebeskind, A., Seidelmann, F., Fogel, J., Franklin, P., & Beltran, J. (2008). Plantar fasciitis and calcaneal spur formation are associated with abductor digiti minimi atrophy on MRI of the foot. *Skeletal Radiology*, 37(6), 505–510.

da Silva Azevedo, A. P., Mezencio, B., Valvassori, R., Mochizuki, L., Amadio, A. C., & Serrao, J. C. (2016). Does "transition shoe" promote an intermediate biomechanical condition compared to running in conventional shoe and in reduced protection condition? *Gait & Posture,* 46, 142-146.

DiGiovanni, B. F., Nawoczenski, D. A., Lintal, M. E., Moore, E. A., Murray, J. C., Wilding, G. E., & Baumhauer, J. F. (2003). Tissue-Specific Plantar Fascia-Stretching Exercise Enhances Outcomes in Patients with Chronic Heel Pain. *The Journal of Bone and Joint Surgery*, 85-A(7), 1270–1277.

Drake, M., Bittenbender, C., & Boyles, R. E. (2011). The short-term effects of treating plantar fasciitis with a temporary custom foot orthosis and stretching. *The Journal of Orthopaedic and Sports Physical Therapy*, 41(4), 221–231.

Eng, J. J., & Pierrynowski, M. R. (1994). The effect of soft foot orthotics on three-dimensional lower-limb kinematics during walking and running. *Physical Therapy*, 74(9), 836–844.

Ferber, R., & Benson, B. (2011). Changes in multi-segment foot biomechanics with a heat-mouldable semi-custom foot orthotic device. *Journal of Foot and Ankle Research*, 4(1), 18–25.

Ferber, R., & Hettinga, B. (2015). A comparison of different over-the-counter foot orthotic devices on multi-segment foot biomechanics. *Prosthetics and Orthotics International*, 1–7.

Fryar, C., Carroll, M., & Ogden, C. (2012). Prevalence of overweight, obesity, and extreme obesity among adults: United States, trends 1960–1962 through 2009–2010. *National Center of Health Statistics.*

Harty, J., Soffe, K., O'Toole, G., & Stephens, M. M. (2005). The Role of Hamstring Tightness in Plantar Fasciitis. *Foot & Ankle International*, 26(12), 1089–1092.

Hohmann, E., Reaburn, P., & Imhoff, A. (2012). Runner's knowledge of their foot type: Do they really know? *The Foot*, 22(3), 205–210.

Jung, D.-Y., Koh, E.-K., & Kwon, O.-Y. (2011). Effect of foot orthoses and short-foot exercise on the cross-sectional area of the abductor halluces muscle in subjects with pes planus: A randomized controlled trial. *Journal of Back and Musculoskeletal Rehabilitation,* 24, 225-231.

Kelly, L. A., Kuitunen, S., Racinais, S., & Cresswell, A. G. (2012). Recruitment of the plantar intrinsic foot muscles with increasing postural demand. *Clinical Biomechanics,* 27, 46-51.

Kirby, K. A. (2016). Understanding Ten Key Biomechanical Functions Of The Plantar Fascia. *Podiatry Today*, 29(7), 1–12.

Knapik, J. J., Trone, D. W., Tchandja, J., & Jones, B. H. (2014). Injury-reduction effectiveness of prescribing running shoes on the basis of foot arch height: Summary of military investigations. *The Journal of Orthopaedic & Sports Physical Therapy*, *44*(10), 805–812.

Kryger, K. O., Jarratt, V., Mitchell, S., & Forrester, S. (2017). Can subjective comfort be used as a measure of plantar pressure in football boots? *Journal of Sports Sciences,* 35(10), 953-959.

Lee, W. E. (2001). Podiatric biomechanics. An historical appraisal and discussion of the Root Model as a Clinical System of Approach in the Present Context of Theoretical Uncertainty. *Clinics in Podiatric Medicine and Surgery*, 18(4), 555–684.

Malisoux, L., Chambon, N., Delattre, N., Gueguen, N., Urhausen, A., & Theisen, D. (2016). Injury risk in runners using standard or motion control shoes: a randomised controlled trial with participant and assessor blinding. *British Journal of Sports Medicine*, 50(8), 481–487.

Martin, R. L., Davenport, T. E., Reischl, S. F., McPoil, T. G., Matheson, J. W., Wukich, D. K., … Godges, J. J. (2014). Heel Pain—Plantar Fasciitis: Revision 2014. *Journal of Orthopaedic & Sports Physical Therapy*, 44(11), A1–A33.

Mckeon, P. O., Hertel, J., Bramble, D., & Davis, I. (2014). The foot core system: a new paradigm for understanding intrinsic foot muscle function. *British Journal of Sports Medicine*, 49, 290–298.

McPoil, T. G., & Hunt, G. C. (1995). Evaluation and management of foot and ankle disorders: present problems and future directions. *The Journal of Orthopaedic and Sports Physical Therapy*, 21(6), 381–388.

Miller, J. E., Nigg, B. M., Liu, W., Stefanyshyn, D. J., & Nurse, M. A. (2000). Influence of foot, leg and shoe characteristics on subjective comfort. *Foot & Ankle International*, 21(9), 759–767.

Mills, K., Blanch, P., & Vicenzino, B. (2011). Influence of contouring and hardness of foot orthoses on ratings of perceived comfort. *Medicine and Science in Sports and Exercise*, 43(8), 1507–1512.

Mulligan, E. P., & Cook, P. G. (2013). Effect of plantar intrinsic muscle training on medial longitudinal arch morphology and dynamic function. *Manual Therapy,* 18, 425-430.

Mündermann, A., Nigg, B. M., Humble, R. N., & Stefanyshyn, D. J. (2003). Orthotic comfort is related to kinematics, kinetics, and EMG in recreational runners. *Medicine and Science in Sports and Exercise*, 35(10), 1710–1719.

Mündermann, A., Nigg, B. M., Stefanyshyn, D. J., & Humble, R. N. (2002). Development of a reliable method to assess footwear comfort during running. *Gait and Posture*, 16(1), 38–45.

Mündermann, A., Stefanyshyn, D. J., & Nigg, B. M. (2001). Relationship between footwear comfort of shoe inserts and anthropometric and sensory factors. *Medicine and Science in Sports and Exercise*, 33(11), 1939–1945.

Pohl, M. B., Hamill, J., & Davis, I. S. (2009). Biomechanical and anatomic factors associated with a history of plantar fasciitis in female runners. *Clinical Journal of Sport Medicine*, 19(5), 372–6.

Protopapas, K., & Perry, S. D. (2020). The effect of a 12-week custom foot orthotic intervention on muscle size and muscle activity of the intrinsic foot muscle of young adults during gait termination. *Clinical Biomechanics,* 78, 1-8.

Ross, M. (2002). Use of the tissue stress model as a paradigm for developing an examination and management plan for a patient with plantar fasciitis. *Journal of the American Podiatric Medical Association*, 92(9), 499–506.

Ryan, M. B., Valiant, G. a, McDonald, K., & Taunton, J. E. (2010). The effect of three different levels of footwear stability on pain outcomes in women runners: a randomised control trial. *British Journal of Sports Medicine*, 45(9), 715–721.

Ryan, M., Elashi, M., Newsham-West, R., & Taunton, J. (2014). Examining injury risk and pain perception in runners using minimalist footwear. *British Journal of Sports Medicine*, 48(16), 1257–1262.

Sackett, D. L., Rosenberg, W. M. C., Gray, J. a M., Haynes, R. B., & Richardson, W. S. (1996). Evidence based medicine: what it is and what it isn't. *British Medical Journal*, 312, 71–72.

Taunton, J. E., Ryan, M. B., Clement, D. B., McKenzie, D. C., Lloyd-Smith, D. R., & Zumbo, B. D. (2003). A prospective study of running injuries: the Vancouver Sun Run "In Training " clinics. *British Journal of Sports Medicine*, 37(1), 239–244.

Made in the USA
Monee, IL
05 November 2026

67383128R00057